Practical Aspects of Blood Administration

Practical Aspects of Blood Administration

Editors

Alice W. Reynolds, (ASCP)SBB
Executive Director
Citrus Regional Blood Center, Inc.
Lakeland, Florida

Del Steckler, RN, BSN
Administrative Director, Transplant Donor Services
American Red Cross
St. Paul, Minnesota

American Association of Blood Banks
Arlington, Virginia
1986

American Association of Blood Banks
1117 North 19th Street, Suite 600
Arlington, Virginia 22209

ISBN No. 0-915355-30-2
First Printing
Printed in the United States

Library of Congress Cataloging-in-Publications Data

Practical aspects of blood administration.

Based on the Practical Aspects of Blood Administration
Technical Workshop held in San Francisco, Calif.,
Nov. 1986.
Includes bibliographies and index.
1. Blood—Transfusion—Congresses. I. Reynolds,
Alice. II. Steckler, Del. III. American Association of
Blood Banks. IV. Practical Aspects of Blood Administra-
tion Technical Workshop (1986 : San Francisco, Calif.)
[DNLM: 1. Blood Banks—congresses. 2. Blood Transfusion
—congresses. WH 460 P895 1986]
RM171.P725 1986   615′.65   86-17470
ISBN 0-915355-30-2

Distributed outside the
United States and Canada by:
S. Karger, AG
Medical and Scientific Publishers
PO Box CH-4009 Basel
Switzerland

Practical Aspects of Blood Administration Technical Workshop

Alice W. Reynolds, (ASCP)SBB, Director
Del Steckler, RN, BSN, Codirector

Committee on Technical/Scientific Workshops

Arthur J. Silvergleid, MD, Chairman

Sandra S. Ellisor, MS, MT(ASCP)SBB
Frances L. Gibbs, MT(ASCP)SBB
Trudell S. Green, MT(ASCP)SBB
W. John Judd, FIMLS, MIBiol
Louise J. Keating, MD
Jerry Kolins, MD
Leo J. McCarthy, MD
Jay E. Menitove, MD
JoAnn Edwards-Moulds, MS, MT(ASCP)SBB
Mary A. Myers, MT(ASCP)SBB
Steven R. Pierce, SBB(ASCP)
Alice W. Reynolds, SBB(ASCP)
Dennis M. Smith, Jr., MD
Del Steckler, RN, BSN
Stephanie Summers, MEd, MT(ASCP)SBB
W. Michael Tregellas, MT(ASCP)SBB
Douglas A. Triplett, MD
Virginia Vengelen-Tyler, MBA, MT(ASCP)SBB
Margaret E. Wallace, MHS, MT(ASCP)SBB

Contents

Foreword

Changes are running rampant throughout the blood banking industry. However, some areas of blood banking are not changing; the desire to provide safe and beneficial blood and blood components to recipients is still of paramount importance. This is the topic of "Practical Aspects of Blood Administration."

The first chapter of this publication deals with recipient consideration in blood administration; this includes pretransfusion care, care during transfusion and posttransfusion care. The second chapter provides critical information on transfusion devices such as filters, needles, catheters, pumps, warmers and compatible solutions. The third chapter answers in-depth questions on the administration of specific blood components. Finally, in Chapter 4, immediate and delayed adverse effects of blood transfusion are addressed.

This manual is designed for the registered nurse administering blood products, the blood bank technologist dispensing blood products and the physician ordering blood products. It is to be used as a reference to answer the numerous questions that arise when blood products are administered. Its purpose is to ensure a safe and efficacious transfusion.

Alice W. Reynolds, (ASCP)SBB
Del Steckler, RN, BSN
Editors

In: Reynolds, AW and Steckler, D, eds.
Practical Aspects of Blood Administration
Arlington, VA: American Association
of Blood Banks, 1986

1

Recipient Considerations

Christina Algiere Kasprisin, RN, MS

*T*HE ABILITY TO SUCCESSFULLY transplant human tissue is becoming more commonplace. Great care is taken in the precise matching of patient and donor. The patient also requires very close monitoring posttransplant. In centers that perform organ transplants, attention to detail is important to ensure that the recipient receives the organ that has the best possible chance of survival.

Blood transfusion is a type of tissue transplant, although it is not always thought of as a transplant. Perhaps it is because this type of transplant has become a common occurrence in most hospitals, or because the transplanted tissue is readily replaced by the donor. In any case, blood transfusions should be delivered with at least the same care and attention to detail as human tissue transplants.

Human errors remain the most common cause of severe acute hemolytic reactions.[1] These can be due to erroneous recipient identification, either at the time the sample is drawn or at the time the component is administered, laboratory error in typing and/or compatibility testing or clerical error. An error in the administration of a red-cell-containing product can cause severe injury and/or death in minutes. For this reason, blood components must be considered by health professionals as some of the most dangerous substances they will ever have to administer.

Indications for Transfusion Therapy

The basic indications for transfusion include the restoration or maintenance of: oxygen-carrying capacity of the blood, blood volume, hemostasis or leukocyte function.

Christina Algiere Kasprisin, RN, MS, Quality Assurance Coordinator-Nursing, Department of Education, Saint Francis Hospital, Tulsa, Oklahoma

1

Anemia

Red blood cells are the treatment of choice in most cases of anemia requiring transfusion. Most surgical cases that require blood can be managed with red blood cells and crystalloids. There is no evidence that any particular hemoglobin level improves the patient's tolerance to surgery or improves wound healing, but many surgical teams have set criteria for presurgical hemoglobin levels. The minimum amount of blood necessary to reach this level should then be infused. While it has been shown that single unit transfusions are more likely to be unnecessary, it is a mistake to use two units of red blood cells to reach a certain hemoglobin level when one unit can accomplish it. The same is true during surgery. The practice of automatically using two units of blood because single unit transfusion is usually contraindicated is wrong if a single unit is sufficient.

Red blood cell transfusions are the component of choice for anemic patients who require transfusion.[2] Transfusing asymptomatic anemic patients is usually unwarranted, since the improvement following transfusion is only temporary and the patient is exposed to all the risks of chronic transfusion. Most patients with chronic anemia will adapt to the anemia. For example, patients with sickle cell anemia will chronically maintain hematocrit levels of 20% and still function normally. The anemic patient with reduced oxygen-carrying capacity will physiologically adapt. In order to deliver adequate oxygen to the tissues, blood flow will increase by an elevation in heart rate and cardiac stroke volume. The patient may feel palpitations and there will be tachycardia, increased pulse pressure, orthopnea, decreased exercise tolerance and dyspnea on exertion. When these compensatory mechanisms no longer function, the patient will develop cardiac failure with venous congestion and pulmonary edema. Transfusion with red cells should be considered when physiologic adaptation begins to fail. However, each patient can tolerate a different hemoglobin level. Usually, patients can tolerate hematocrits of 25% before having symptoms of orthopnea, excessive weakness and eventually cardiac failure. Patients with acute loss of red blood cells will usually be symptomatic at higher laboratory values than individuals with slow, chronic loss of red cells. Children can usually tolerate lower levels than adults. Ten ml/kg body weight of red cells will raise the hemoglobin by 3 g/dl.[3]

When the patient is symptomatic, several things can be done to increase patient safety and comfort while reducing the individual's energy expenditure. These interventions may allow time for identification of the cause of the anemia, if intervention is indicated, and for the initiation of medical rather than transfusion therapy. The decreased oxygen-carrying capacity of the blood will result in symptomatic activity intolerance. Attention should be directed at minimizing the anemic individual's energy expenditure. This can be done by providing assistance for daily activities, ensuring a rest period, and administering oxygen when prescribed by the physician.

Blood Volume Replacement

Restoration of circulating blood volume is a controversial issue in medicine. In acute massive hemorrhage, the colloid-crystalloid debate continues. Current evidence suggests that rapid infusion of normal saline or lactated Ringer's (2 liters initially) will allow time for typing and screening of the patient's blood. A blood loss of 1–1.5 liters can usually be tolerated without requiring blood replacement if the patient's blood volume is maintained with crystalloids, but each case must be individualized.[4] Rapid blood loss in an unstable, fragile patient may justify intervening with blood transfusion at an earlier point.

The physiologic response to an acute bleeding episode depends on the severity of the hemorrhage. When the blood loss equals 10–15% of the total blood volume, there are minimal symptoms. The body moves fluid from the extracellular space into the vasculature. There is also a contraction of the great veins. When the blood loss reaches 20%, symptoms are still limited. Tachycardia is usually present on exertion and there may be slight orthostatic hypotension. A blood loss of 30% requires considerably greater use of compensatory mechanisms. Orthostatic hypotension and tachycardia on exertion are present but the rising blood pressure and pulse may still be normal, especially if the patient is in a supine position. Blood flow to the skin and muscles is decreased and the arterioles are constricted. Glycolysis and lipolysis are increased with metabolic acidosis and compensatory respiratory alkalosis. Urinary output decreases and the patient is thirsty. The patient is markedly symptomatic when the blood loss reaches 40%. The resting blood pressure and central venous pressure are low. The patient demonstrates air hunger, the skin is clammy and the pulse is thready. Consciousness is altered. The patient becomes shocky when the blood loss reaches 50% and death is imminent if treatment is not begun quickly.[5]

Hemostasis

Platelets are the cellular component of the clotting mechanism. Thrombocytopenic patients and patients with abnormal platelet function are at risk of severe hemorrhagic episodes. Platelets are used both prophylactically and therapeutically in these patients. The effectiveness of platelet transfusion in thrombocytopenic patients depends on several factors. The normal platelet count is 250,000–400,000/mm³. Severe spontaneous bleeding due to thrombocytopenia usually does not occur unless the count is below 25,000/mm³. Patients with platelet counts of less than 75,000–100,000/mm³ are at risk if they require any surgical intervention.

Whether platelets should be used in an individual case depends on several factors. The first consideration is the patient's platelet count. Although spontaneous bleeding usually does not occur until the count is less than 25,000/mm³, prophylactic platelet transfusion is usually not necessary until the count is less than 5–10,000/mm³. Patients recovering from bone marrow suppression are more likely to have younger, more functional platelets and may have less tendency to bleed than a patient whose platelet count is dropping because of a nonfunctioning marrow.[6] When the marrow stops producing platelets due to drugs, aplasia or neoplasm, the platelets continue in the circulation until they die. These older platelets are less functional. Therefore, a patient with a recovering bone marrow will usually have fewer bleeding problems than a patient with a failing marrow, even when both have the same platelet count.

Patients who are destroying their platelets due to antibody (such as idiopathic thrombocytopenic purpura), splenomegaly, intravascular coagulation, thrombotic thrombocytopenic purpura and other diseases usually do not have an increase in platelet count following transfusion. Because of the short life span of platelets transfused into these patients, prophylactic platelet transfusion is not beneficial and transfusion is limited in these patients to the treatment of significant hemorrhages.

Fresh frozen plasma (FFP) is the liquid portion of the blood frozen within a few hours of the time of collection. All the protein coagulation factors are preserved, including the labile Factors V, VIII and XI. The principal use of FFP is supplying clotting factors, particularly these labile factors. FFP is occasionally used as a volume expander and protein source, but crystalloids, albumin or plasma protein fraction can usually be substituted without incurring the risk of hepatitis and other transfusion-transmitted infections. It has also been used to supply opsonins (proteins such as immunoglobulins, complement and fibronectin that help phagocytosis) in septic neonates and immunodeficient patients, but there has been little research to prove its value for this purpose.[7]

The labile clotting Factors V, VIII and XI deteriorate rapidly and whole blood cannot supply these factors unless it is very fresh. Since FFP can be stored frozen for 1 year, it is more suitable as a

supply of coagulation factors; also, it does not add other components, such as red cells, that the patient may not need. Some of the
clotting factors can be supplied in a more concentrated form, and
the use of these products will be discussed in Chapter 3.

Plasma components should not be used to replace clotting factors in nonemergencies when the patient is deficient in the vitamin
K dependent clotting Factors II, VII, IX and X, when the clotting
defect can be corrected with vitamin K. When it is necessary to
supply these factors, FFP, liquid plasma or pooled concentrate can
be used.

In patients who have difficulty with hemostasis due to either
platelet dysfunction or clotting factor disturbance, safety needs are
of increasing importance. These individuals who may not be clinically symptomatic should be carefully taught and observed to maintain the fragile hemostatic balance. These measures include: no
intramuscular or subcutaneous injections, careful selection of venipuncture site and appropriate precautions when blood samples
must be obtained and, above all, careful attention to minimize any
trauma.

Neutropenia

Granulocytes are the cellular component of the blood that is needed
to help fight bacterial infections. Patients with severe granulocytopenia, ie, leukemia, aplastic anemia and patients on cancer chemotherapy, have a significant risk of life-threatening bacterial infections. The criteria for the use of granulocyte transfusions are[8]:
1. Granulocytopenia less than 1000/μl but usually less than 500/
    μl
2. Documented bacterial infection
3. A lack of response to appropriate antibiotic therapy for at least
    24–72 hours after infection with an antibiotic-resistant organ-
    ism
4. A bone marrow that is not expected to recover within a reason-
    able period of time but a case in which there is some expec-
    tation for a reasonable survival

Several measures can be instituted for the granulocytopenic
patient. These include avoidance of individuals who may be sick
and scrupulous attention to aseptic technique for any invasive
procedures.

Volunteer Blood Supply

Volunteer donors come to a blood center because they want to
give blood. This premise is considered essential in maintaining a

safe, adequate blood supply. With the growth of blood banking since the close of World War II, numerous strategies have been used to ensure an adequate blood supply. These have included paying the donor, offering other incentives, and using nonincentive programs. Studies have verified that the use of commercial donors has an increased risk of hepatitis compared with a volunteer donor population. The Transfusion-Transmitted Virus Study (TTVS)[9] demonstrated that the relative risk of hepatitis from community service blood banks was 6.4% compared with 15.7% for centers that offered replacement units and 38.5% for those patients receiving only commercial blood.

This study also indicated a geographic variance in the risk of transfusion-associated hepatitis when only community service agencies were used. Houston had the highest rate, followed by Los Angeles and New York, with the lowest risk of hepatitis in St. Louis. This type of geographical variance is now being seen in the screening of blood donors for HTLV-III.[10]

Health professionals should do all that is possible to ensure a volunteer blood supply. The volunteer presumably has no motive for blood donation except the desire to perform a community service. The volunteer blood supply is currently at risk due to the recently surfaced fear of Acquired Immune Deficiency Syndrome (AIDS). Many people are requesting/demanding that they receive blood components only from family members or friends. Studies are in progress to determine if these "directed donations" have any lower risk of disease transmission than a totally volunteer donor system. It has been proposed that individuals who may be members of a risk group are forced by peer pressure into donating, for fear of being identified as risk group members. In addition, individuals who are regular blood donors may cease donating so that they will be eligible to donate if a relative or friend requires a transfusion.

Patients having elective surgery should be informed about the feasibility of autologous transfusion. Currently, red cells can be stored in the liquid state for 42 days. This allows the patient to predeposit 2 or more units that can be reinfused at the time of surgery, if needed. In addition, if blood is withdrawn 5 to 7 days before surgery, the patient's rate of red cell production will be increased at the time of surgery.

Pretransfusion Care

It is the responsibility of the physician to order blood components for administration to the patient. Specific criteria have been established to guide physicians in the use of blood components.[11] Transfusion therapy has many life-saving benefits, but it also has many attendant risks, including the possibility of disease transmission, transfusion reactions and death due to a severe reaction or human error. For these reasons, blood components must only be used when the benefits of transfusion outweigh any of the associated risks.

Once the decision to transfuse has been made, the transfusion team must do everything possible to ensure that the patient will receive the maximal benefit of transfusion while minimizing the attendant risks. Careful attention to detail will help prevent the most frequent cause of transfusion mishap—human error.

Preparing the Recipient

The physician's order should be verified and compared with both the patient's clinical status and laboratory values. If there is any question about the necessity for transfusion, it must be clarified with the physician before the transfusion is given. The initial order must specify the desired component, the quantity to be infused and any special circumstances that need to be considered.

Religious Beliefs

During the pretransfusion preparation, an additional check should be done to verify that the patient's religious beliefs do not prohibit blood component therapy. While the majority of organized religions do not prohibit the use of blood products by their members when a medical need exists, the Jehovah's Witnesses and Christian Scientists include in their teachings prohibitions against transfusion therapy. However, believers of these and other faiths may have modified their position on blood component therapy. Therefore, all patients should be given the opportunity to discuss their beliefs regarding blood transfusion without generalizations being made.

If a child requires blood component therapy and the parents refuse based on religious beliefs, the physician may be able to obtain a court order to allow the transfusion to occur. This is an ethical dilemma that should be explored in advance. If the court allows the transfusion to take place, the parents may be either relieved that their child was saved without their having to compromise their religious beliefs or angered to the point of rejecting the child, since, in their religion, the child now has no chance for salvation.[12]

Table 1-1. Patient Education: Signs of a Transfusion Reaction

Vague uneasy feeling
Onset of pain (especially IV site, back, chest)
Breathing difficulties
Chills/flush
Nausea/dizziness
Rash
Dark or red urine

Patient Education

The patient's understanding of the procedure should be assessed. Discussion with the patient should cover the complete sequence of events, including the crossmatch, IV line and activity limitations, if any. To minimize the risks of component therapy, the patient and/or family should be taught the signs and symptoms that may be associated with a complication of component therapy. Warning signs are listed in Table 1-1. If explained too graphically, the patient may have symptoms of a reaction before the transfusion is even begun. The patient should be asked to report any "different" sensations after the tranfusion has been initiated. When the patient is a young child or disoriented adult, the family can be instructed and asked to observe for any signs of an untoward reaction. The informed patient and family can aid in the early detection of problems.

Informed Consent

Prior to ordering the necessary blood components, the physician will discuss the need for transfusion with the patient. The recipient must be alerted to the benefits and risks of component therapy, alternative therapies, if any, and the risks, if the patient chooses against therapy. Documentation that the patient understands the benefits and risks of transfusion therapy should be in the medical record. Legally competent adults are capable of reviewing this information, making a decision about therapy and giving consent for the transfusion. If the adult is unable to give consent because of mental status or physical condition, then next of kin, a legal guardian or the court must be provided with the information to provide an informed consent.

Pediatric transfusions pose a unique set of circumstances. Most states consider 18 as the age at which a child becomes an adult. An adolescent is considered emancipated if marrried, pregnant, a member of the armed services or has been deserted by the parents.

Emancipated adolescents are considered capable of deciding the course of their therapy.

Even though pediatric patients are not capable of providing a legal informed consent for therapy, they should be included in the discussion. The therapy should be explàined in terms that they can understand. Children over the age of 7 have been judged to be capable of providing assent for therapy. The child's cooperation should be enlisted and the child asked to sign the consent form along with the parents or legal guardian. Adolescents aged 15 and above have been judged competent to provide their own consent for therapy. This rule, known as the mature minor precedent, states that the older adolescent can weigh the benefits and risks of therapy and give a true informed consent.[13]

Laboratory Interface

While the transfusionist is readying the patient, the laboratory can be preparing the blood component necessary for transfusion. Hospital policy usually will dictate the procedure required for obtaining the patient specimen. A properly labeled requisition designating the quantity and type of component is mandatory. The patient's name and identifying hospital number must also be included. A blood specimen from the intended recipient is required for type and screen.[14 (p 195)]

Attention to detail is absolutely essential as this first step is performed. Before obtaining the blood specimens for typing, the phlebotomist should ask patients to identify themselves and check the hospital identification bracelet. These should be checked against the laboratory requisition. Asking patients to spell their name can be used as an additional safeguard. The phlebotomist should never state the patient's name and wait for a response. Many patients will answer affirmatively to names other than their own if they are confused or disoriented. If patients cannot identify themselves, family members, if present, can be asked to verify the patient's identity. Many institutions utilize special blood identification systems. A new number is assigned to each patient and this number is attached to the specimen being sent to the laboratory. This same number is then affixed to the blood components that are being readied for transfusion to the patient. When the component is ready to be infused, the second identification system provides a double check for patient identity. These systems are not foolproof—human errors can and do still occur.

The specimen tube must be labeled before it leaves the patient's bedside. Once the crossmatch specimen has been obtained, the laboratory can then identify compatible blood components for this patient. When the situation is emergent, the laboratory should be notified when the order is written. This will inform all departments that expediency is required. The laboratory usually notifies the nursing unit when the prescribed component is available or if there is a problem in identifying compatible blood for the patient.

The transfusionist should communicate with the blood bank regarding when the blood component will be available. If the patient has irregular antibodies, more time may be required to locate blood components that are negative for the corresponding antigen. In addition, special processing time may be required for thawing fresh frozen plasma, washing red cells or obtaining HLA-compatible products. The patient should be kept informed regarding the time frame that is anticipated.

Preparation of the Patient

The first preparations for component therapy include ensuring adequate venous access and obtaining baseline vital signs. For the transfusion of red cell products, a large-gauge needle is preferred. For adults, an 18- or 19-gauge needle is recommended. This size needle provides for a good rate of flow without undue discomfort for the patient. In the chronically transfused or pediatric patient where adequate venous access is difficult to maintain, the largest possible needle should be used. Red cells can be safely administered through 23- to 25-gauge needles, but the flow rate will be slower.[15] Non-red-cell-containing blood products such as platelets, FFP, albumin and cryoprecipitate can be rapidly administered through small-gauge needles.

When an intravenous line is being started, several factors should be considered. In adults, when possible, the nondominant hand should be used. This allows the patient the comfort of having the dominant hand free from restraint. In young children who are not yet walking, the feet can be used. This allows their hands free to explore the environment. Once the child is walking, then the non-dominant hand should be considered. An armboard may be necessary to stabilize the extremity. When a pre-existing intravenous site will be utilized, the patency of the line should be assessed. This includes examining the infusion site for signs of swelling, redness, pain, differences in color or slowed infusion rate. A blood return in the tubing does not always ensure that the venous access is adequate.

A Y-type blood administration set can be used for red cell administration. These sets have an in-line filter (approximately 170 micron) that is necessary to remove fibrin clots and other large aggregates from blood components. When the patient will be massively transfused, then a microaggregate filter should be used. If a Y-type administration set is being used, normal saline can be aseptically introduced into the unit of red cells to decrease the viscosity. Newer additive solutions used in red cell preparations may make this unnecessary.

The administration set should be primed with normal saline. This is the preferred solution for blood component administration. Prolonged contact between red cells and solutions containing dextrose can result in a loss of water from the red cell and subsequent destruction. Solutions containing calcium, such as lactated Ringer's have been shown to interfere with the anticoagulant used in the red blood cells.[16]

The final step before initiating transfusion therapy should be a thorough assessment of the patient. Temperature, pulse, respiration and blood pressure should be monitored just prior to initiating the transfusion. These will provide a baseline measurement against which any changes during the transfusion can be compared. Measurements of all vital signs should be recorded in the patient record and be available for comparison. The recipient should also be questioned about any symptoms such as chills, itching, rashes, muscle aches or difficulty breathing that may later be mistaken for a transfusion reaction.

Patient Comfort

A non-emergent transfusion of red cells will take about 1-½ to 2 hours to infuse. The patient should be assisted to the bathroom and made comfortable before the transfusion is begun. This will allow fewer manipulations of the blood and tubing during the course of administration. Patients with a history of febrile nonhemolytic transfusion reactions may be premedicated with an antipyretic such as acetaminophen before the transfusion. Since aspirin interferes with platelet function, patients who may have a secondary clotting disturbance should not receive aspirin-containing products for fever control. Washed red blood cells may also be used for patients with a history of febrile and allergic transfusion reactions.

Initiating the Transfusion

The procedure for obtaining the blood component from the hospital blood bank and delivering it to the patient for transfusion varies in each institution. Essential guidelines that must be adhered to, regardless of the procedure, include: start of infusion within 30 minutes of the time the component is released from the blood bank, proper identification of the blood component and the recip-

Table 1-2. Blood Component and Recipient Identification

Component
Physician order—component received
ABO-Rh type—identical on label and compatibility tag
Expiration date

Recipient
ABO-Rh type—compatible with donor
Name and hospital number identical to compatibility tag

ient and careful handling of the blood component while it is in transit. If the transfusion is delayed more than 30 minutes, the component should be returned to the blood bank for proper storage.

The final step of preparation is the proper identification of the blood component and the recipient. Regardless of how many times the transfusionist has interacted with the patient, the appropriate checks must be done. Table 1-2 lists the items that must be verified before the transfusion is initiated. It should be remembered that human errors are the leading cause of death in transfusion therapy. Those hospital areas in which the greatest number of deaths occur are the operating rooms and the intensive care units. Patients who are unable to identify themselves are at greatest risk.[17]

Because of the antigenicity of red cells, transfusions containing red cells are most likely to produce severe reactions. Observation of the patient during the initial part of the transfusion is recommended. For adult patients, it is recommended that the first 50 ml be infused over 15 minutes. In pediatric patients, $\frac{1}{5}$ of the volume should be infused over this time period. With red cell transfusions, any severe reactions will usually occur during the transfusion of this small volume, and the ready availability of help can minimize the adverse effects of a severe transfusion reaction. Once this initial period is safely over, the rate of flow can be increased to complete the transfusion within 1-$\frac{1}{2}$ to 2 hours. The patient's vital signs should be monitored at the end of the first 15 minutes and then periodically throughout the transfusion.

Infusion Pumps

Infusion control devices are becoming more common in acute care institutions. The research evidence indicates that there is little if any increased hemolysis secondary to use of most infusion pumps. The manufacturer's literature will provide detailed information on the suitability of any particular infusion pump for transfusing blood components.

Medications

Drugs should never be mixed with the blood component to be administered. Besides the indeterminate effect the medication may have on the blood component, if a reaction occurs, it would be difficult to ascertain whether the drug or the blood component was responsible for the adverse effect. Also, if the transfusion is interrupted for any reason, it would be impossible to calculate the amount of drug the patient received. If the patient will require intravenous drugs during the course of the transfusion, a separate intravenous line should be started for the blood. In this manner, the patient can receive the therapeutic effects of the blood component as well as the medications.

Duration of Transfusion

The transfusion of red cell products should be completed in 4 hours or less. In patients with compromised cardiovascular systems or inadequate venous access, where it is anticipated that the transfusion cannot be completed in 4 hours, the blood bank should be notified of the anticipated difficulty. The unit of blood can be subdivided prior to the transfusion and half can remain under controlled conditions while the patient receives the first half. This unit splitting can also be done for pediatric patients who will require smaller volume transfusions over a period of several days. The individual portions of the unit can be released for transfusion while the remainder is safely stored. This method reduces the amount of foreign blood to which the child is exposed. A new crossmatch specimen is required if more than 2 days elapse.[14 (p 287)]

Maintenance of Transfusion

If the blood component is infusing too slowly, the tranfusionist should investigate the probable causes. The first area that should be checked is the intravenous access. The site should be assessed for signs of infiltration. If the line is no longer patent, then a new venous access should be started as soon as possible. When the component is infusing by gravity, raising the height of the blood container should increase the rate of flow. Gently massaging the unit may aid by resuspending the red cells. Finally, the filter in the administration set may become clogged with debris. Whenever this occurs, the tubing should be changed.

Multiple Unit Transfusions

Often, a patient will receive two or more units of red cells or other blood components. Definitive studies have not been done on the amount of time or the number of units that can be infused through one administration set. Product literature suggests that two to four units can be infused through one set. Some institutions require that both the administration set and blood component not remain in use longer than 4 hours. The tubing should be checked frequently to ensure that a clogged filter will be detected early. Once the tubing has been used, it should not remain connected to the patient for prolonged periods of time.

Termination of the Transfusion

Completion of Transfusion

When the prescribed volume of blood component has been infused, then the transfusion can be terminated. If the intravenous line was established solely for purposes of the transfusion, it can be discontinued. The patient's maintenance solution should be restarted with new intravenous lines.

The patient must be thoroughly assessed and temperature, pulse, respiration and blood pressure monitored. This information should be documented in the patient's medical record. Some reactions may occur after the completion of the transfusion. The patient should be reminded to report any signs or symptoms.

The blood container and administration set must be disposed of according to the institution policy. Blood products should be handled as if they have the potential for disease transmission. The used equipment must be carefully handled and packaged to protect other members of the health-care team.

Discharge Instructions

The patient should be observed at the completion of the component therapy. Vital signs should be taken and recorded. Signs and symptoms of a transfusion reaction should again be reviewed with the patient/family. They should also be alerted to the possibility of delayed transfusion reactions.

Signs of Transfusion Reactions

The pathophysiology and definitive treatment of transfusion reactions will be discussed later in Chapter 4. Since the possibility of a transfusion reaction is always present, the responsibility for recognition and initial intervention rests with the transfusionist. See Table 1-3.

Febrile or allergic reactions may occur with fever and chills in the same manner as a severe hemolytic reaction. For this reason, any adverse change in the patient's condition should be considered a possible symptom of a transfusion reaction and evaluated.

Institutional policy will dictate the exact sequence of events that must take place when a transfusion reaction is suspected. However, the essential elements are universal: 1) the transfusion should be immediately halted, 2) the intravenous access should be kept patent for treatment if necessary and 3) the responsible physician must be notified to evaluate the patient.

Individuals who have had multiple transfusion or who have had numerous pregnancies are at greatest risk for febrile transfusion reactions. A patient who has had one febrile transfusion reaction is at greater risk for subsequent reactions. Some physicians premedicate these patients at high risk with acetaminophen. This medication is given in an attempt to maintain patient comfort in the event of a reaction. Despite the medication, the patient may still have a severe reaction; therefore, premedication does not eliminate the need for an astute observer.

When a severe reaction is suspected, then the administration set should be changed. This allows the 10–15 ml of blood remaining in the tubing to be discarded rather than infused into the patient.

The presenting signs and symptoms, the patient status and the actions of the involved health professional should be carefully documented.

Outpatient Transfusion Therapy

Changes in the health-care system are prompting an increasing use of outpatient services. Many acute care institutions and home health agencies have added outpatient transfusion therapy to the services they provide. The procedures and requirements for safe, effective transfusion therapy do not change if the patient is an outpatient. All of the appropriate blood component and patient identification checks must be done. The major difference is that the patient will not have prolonged contact with a health professional after the transfusion is completed.

Table 1-3.   Care of the Patient Receiving Blood Transfusions

Complication	Signs/Symptoms	Precautions/Nursing Responsibilities
Immediate reactions		
Hemolytic reactions (most severe type, but rare) Incompatible blood Intradonor incompatibility in multiple transfusions	Chills Shaking Fever Pain at needle site and along venous tract Nausea/vomiting Sensation of tightness in chest Red or black urine Headache Flank pain If progressive, signs of shock and/or renal failure	Positively identify donor and recipient blood types and groups before transfusion is begun, verify with one other nurse or physician Transfuse blood slowly for first 15 to 20 minutes and/or initial ⅕ volume of blood; remain with patient In event of signs or symptoms, stop transfusion immediately, maintain patent intravenous line, and notify physician Save donor blood to recross-match with patient's blood Monitor blood pressure for shock Insert urinary catheter and monitor hourly outputs Send sample of patient's blood and urine to laboratory for presence of hemoglobin (indicates intravascular hemolysis) Observe for signs of hemorrhage resulting from disseminated intravascular coagulation (DIC) Support medical therapies to reverse shock

Cause	Signs/Symptoms	Considerations
Febrile reactions Leukocyte or platelet antibodies Plasma protein antibodies	Fever Chills	May give acetaminophen or antihistamines for prophylaxis Use of leukocyte-poor red blood cells is less likely to cause reaction Stop transfusion immediately, report to physician for evaluation
Allergic reactions—recipient reacts to allergens in donor's blood	Urticaria Flushing Asthmatic wheezing Laryngeal edema	Give antihistamines for prophylaxis to individuals with a tendency toward allergic reactions Stop transfusions immediately Epinephrine may be used for wheezing or anaphylactic reaction
Circulatory overload Too rapid transfusion (even if small quantity) Excessive quantity of blood transfused (even if slowly)	Precordial plan Dyspnea Rales Cyanosis Dry cough Distended neck veins	Transfuse blood slowly Prevent overload by using packed red blood cells or administering divided amounts of blood Use infusion pump to regulate and maintain flow rate If signs of overload, stop transfusion immediately Place patient in semi-Fowler position to increase venous resistance
Air emboli—may occur when blood is transfused under pressure	Sudden difficulty in breathing Sharp pain in chest Apprehension	When infusing blood under pressure before container is empty If air is observed in tubing, clamp tubing

Table 1-3. Care of the Patient Receiving Blood Transfusions—Continued

Complication	Signs/Symptoms	Precautions/Nursing Responsibilities
		immediately below air bubble, clear tubing of air by aspirating air with syringe or disconnecting tubing and allowing blood to flow until air has escaped
Delayed hemolytic reaction	Destruction of red blood cells and fever 5 to 10 days after transfusion	Observe for posttransfusion anemia and decreasing benefit from successive transfusions
Hypothermia	Chills Low temperature Irregular heart rate Possible cardiac arrest	Allow blood to warm at room temperature (less than 1 hour) Use an electric warming coil to rapidly warm blood Take temperature if patient complains of chills; if subnormal, stop transfusion
Electrolyte disturbances Hyperkalemia (only in massive transfusions or in patients with renal problems)	Nausea, diarrhea Muscular weakness Flaccid paralysis Paresthesia of extremities Bradycardia Apprehension Cardiac arrest	Use washed red blood cells or fresh blood if patient at risk

"Citrate" intoxication (hypocalcemia)	Tingling in fingers Tetany Muscular cramps Carpopedal spasm Hyperactive reflexes Convulsions Laryngeal spasm Respiratory arrest	Infuse blood slowly (citrate reaction less likely to occur) If signs of tetany occur, clamp tubing immediately, maintain patent intravenous line, and notify physician
Delayed reactions Transmission of infection Hepatitis AIDS Malaria Syphilis Bacteria or viruses Other	Signs of infection after transfusion, for example, jaundice from hepatitis Bacterial or toxin contamination—high fever, severe headache or substernal pain, hypotension, intense flushing, vomiting/diarrhea	Blood is tested for HBsAg (hepatitis B), syphilis and in most centers HTLV-III (AIDS); positive units are destroyed. Individuals at risk for carrying certain viruses are deferred from donation Report any sign of infection, and if occurring during transfusion, stop transfusion immediately, send sample for culture and sensitivity tests, and notify physician
Alloimmunization (antibody formation)	Increased risk of hemolytic, febrile and allergic reactions	Occurs in patients receiving multiple transfusions Use limited number of donors Observe carefully for signs of reactions

Reproduced (adapted) with permission from Whaley LR and Wong L. Nursing care of infants and children. 2nd ed. St. Louis: The C. V. Mosby Co., 1983.[18]

References

1. Myhre BA. Fatalities from blood transfusion. JAMA 1980; 244:1333–5.
2. Snyder EL, ed. Blood transfusion therapy: A physician's handbook. Arlington, VA: American Association of Blood Banks, 1983:9.
3. Luban NLC. Blood groups and blood component transfusion. In: Miller DR, Baehner RL, McMillan CW, eds. Blood diseases of infancy and childhood. St. Louis: The CV Mosby Co., 1984:68.
4. Beckwith N, Carriere SR. Fluid resuscitation in trauma: An update. J Emer Nsg 1985;11:293–9.
5. Collins JA. The pathophysiology of hemorrhagic shock. In: Collins JA, Murawski K, Shafer AW, eds. Massive transfusion in surgery and trauma. New York: AR Liss, 1982:5–29.
6. Johnston MFM. Blood component therapy. In: Rutman RC, Miller WV, eds. Transfusion therapy principles and procedures, 2nd ed. Rockville, MD: Aspen Publications, 1985:29–40.
7. Oberman HA. Uses and abuses of fresh frozen plasma. In: Garratty A, ed. Current concepts in transfusion therapy. Arlington, VA: American Association of Blood Banks, 1985:109–24.
8. Kasprisin DO, Ilangovan S, Salmassi S. Indications for granulocyte transfusions. Plasma Ther Transfus Technol 1982;3:429–38.
9. Hollinger FB, Mosley JW, Szmuness W, et al. Non-A, non-B hepatitis following blood transfusion: Risk factors associated with donor characteristics. In: Viral hepatitis. 1981 International Symposium. Philadelphia: The Franklin Institute Press, 1981:361–76.
10. Schorr JB, Berkowitz A, Cumming PD, Katz AJ, Sandler SG. Prevalence of HTLV-III antibody in American blood donors. N Engl J Med 1986;313:384–5.
11. Simpson MB. Audit criteria for transfusion practices. In: Wallas CH, Muller VH, eds. The hospital transfusion committee. Arlington, VA: American Association of Blood Banks, 1982:21–60.
12. Holder AR. Parents, courts, and refusal of treatment. J Pediatr 1983;103:515–21.
13. Leikin SL. Minors' assent or dissent to medical treatment. J Pediatr 1983;102:169–76.
14. Widmann FK, ed. Technical manual. 9th ed. Arlington, VA: American Association of Blood Banks, 1985.

15. Butch SH, Coltre MA. Techniques of transfusion. In: Kasprisin DO, Luban NLC, eds. Pediatric transfusion medicine. Boca Raton, FL: CRC Press (in press).
16. Ryden SE, Oberman HA. Compatibility of common intravenous solutions with CPD blood. Transfusion 1975;15:250–5.
17. Schmidt PJ. Transfusion mortality with specific reference to surgical and intensive care facilities. AORN J 1981;34:1114–22.
18. Whaley LR, Wong DL. Nursing care of infants and children, 2nd ed. St. Louis: The CV Mosby Co, 1983.

In: Reynolds, AW and Steckler, D, eds.
Practical Aspects of Blood Administration
Arlington, VA: American Association
of Blood Banks, 1986

2

Transfusion Devices

Roberta D. Schell, RN

*M*ANY DEVICES EXIST FOR the transfusion of blood and blood products. The proper use of these devices and the use of compatible solutions are two critical steps in the delivery of safe and beneficial blood and blood components to the recipient. This chapter will explore debris formations, the types of filters and their appropriate use, compatible solutions for use with blood and blood components, the types of blood warmers and pumps available, needle and catheter selection as well as calculation of flow rates.

Filtration

The American Association of Blood Banks' *Standards* states that "blood and blood components shall be maintained in a controlled environment at optimal temperatures until released for transfusion. They must be transfused through a sterile, pyrogen-free transfusion set which has a filter capable of retaining particles potentially harmful to the recipient."[1] (p 30) The characteristics of a good blood filter[2] should include the ability to:

1. Remove all damaging particles from the blood, hence the largest particles passed must not occlude critical vasculature
2. Maintain a negligible resistance to flow
3. Exhibit minimal trauma to blood, ie, it must not remove viable blood components
4. Maintain a minimal flow velocity with low flow turbulence
5. Be easily primed
6. Have a low priming volume

Roberta D. Schell, RN, Provider Relations Representative, American Medical International/Group Health Service, Beverly Hills, California

Debris Formation

The idea that a filter had to be incorporated into the drip chamber of a set resulted from the realization by early blood bankers that clots formed in bank blood during storage. The clotting was of a gross nature and was first seen as a plug in the catheters. This debris formation is due to many factors. Inadequate mixing during collection along with storage at 1 C contribute to debris formation. The accumulation of debris begins within 2 to 24 hours after collection with the length of storage time being critical to the amount of debris.[3-5]

Light[3,6] and electron microscopy studies have shown that microaggregates are composed largely of degenerating platelets, granulocytes, denatured proteins, fibrin strands and other debris. They vary in size from 10 to more than 200 microns in diameter.

The formation of microaggregates in stored blood occurs because the blood has been removed from the usual cell replacement and cell removal processes of the body. The preservation of the blood is directed primarily at the red blood cells (RBCs), whose life span in the body is 100 to 120 days. The other cellular components have much shorter life spans, ranging from a few days for platelets to 21 days for lymphocytes.

The formation of microaggregates begins during the first 24 hours of storage. During the first few days of storage, the microaggregates consist almost entirely of degenerating platelets. Toward the end of the first week of storage, degenerating granulocytes also begin to aggregate and join the platelet aggregates. For the duration of storage, the number of viable leukocytes declines steadily, with an increasing amount of debris formation.

Microaggregate formation is also affected by the anticoagulant used to store the blood. Heparin causes microaggregates to form within hours of collection. In CPD (citrate, phosphate, dextrose) and CPDA-1 (citrate, phosphate, dextrose, adenine-1), the more common anticoagulants in current use, microaggregate formation begins within the first several days after collection and continues throughout the duration of storage. The shelf life of CPD blood is 21 days; the shelf life of CPDA-1 blood is 35 days.

There are two newly approved blood additive systems designed to extend the storage of red blood cells, which also may improve plasma and platelet yields. One of these systems is Nutricel™, made by Cutter Biological Division of Miles Laboratories, with a 42-day shelf life for RBCs. The other is Adsol™, produced by Fenwal Division of Travenol Laboratories, with a 49-day outdate for RBCs. The platelets and plasma products collected using these systems are stored in CPD. Although there is at this time no documentation on the number of microaggregates that form in these solutions, it is assumed that, as in other anticoagulants, microaggregates do form.

Standard Clot Screen Filters

Initial attempts at filtration included the use of stainless steel mesh, glass beads, bakelite, rayon and gauze. Ultimately, the standard clot screen, with pores of 170–230 microns, was incorporated into blood administration sets. Commercial filters come with myriad features to meet specific needs required in various areas of transfusion practice.

If blood or a blood component is the only substance to be infused, a straight-line blood administration set is appropriate. This straight-line set is offered in two different ways. The filter is either housed inside the drip chamber or as a set with a separate filter and drip chamber. With either type of set, the blood filter should be completely immersed in blood for optimum utilization of its surface area.

The immersion of the filter is accomplished by moving the roller clamp as close to the drip chamber as possible and closing it. The protective cap is removed from the spike, and the port at the top of the blood bag is exposed as the tabs are pulled back. The port should never be touched as it would then be contaminated. Next, the spike is inserted into the port with a twisting motion, with care to avoid piercing the bag with the spike. Puncturing of the blood bag would mean discarding the unit and replacing that unit of blood with another. After the spike is inserted, the set is then hung.

When a straight-line set with a separate filter and drip chamber is used, the filter is filled with blood by squeezing the drip chamber. Squeezing the filter will cause it to rupture. When a set with a combination drip chamber/filter is used, the chamber is filled by squeezing it directly. Once the filter set is primed, the roller clamp is opened and the tubing is primed. Care must be taken to expel all the air. The filter is tapped to dislodge any trapped air bubbles.

A Y-set is used if a component requires dilution to reduce viscosity, if saline is needed to begin the infusion or if the transfusion is to be followed by another intravenous solution or blood component.

Before beginning the procedure, all clamps on the Y-set should be closed: the main flow rate clamp, the clamp on the blood line (with the unvented tubing) and the clamp on the saline solution line (with the vented tubing). Two units of a blood component should not be attached to a Y-tubing set for sequential transfusion.

Next, the spike is uncapped on the saline solution line. When using a glass bottle, the port of the saline solution container is swabbed with alcohol, and the spike is inserted into the container. The cap is removed from the blood line spike and the blood bag ports are exposed as the two tabs at the top of the bag are pulled back. The port should not be contaminated by human touch. The bag is spiked and the entire Y-set is hung on the IV pole. The saline solution line clamp is opened and the combination drip chamber is squeezed until it is half full. The needle adapter cover is removed and the main flow rate clamp is opened to prime the tubing. Both clamps are then closed and the needle adapter is recapped. The blood line clamp is opened and the combination drip chamber/ filter on the Y-set is squeezed until the filter is completely immersed in blood. Preparing both the straight-line set and/or the Y-set in the above-described fashion ensures readiness to proceed with the transfusion.

These standard clot screen filters can be used to infuse two to four units of blood, depending upon the manufacturer, the age of the blood and the type of blood component. Accumulation of debris results in a slower flow rate and the ultimate necessity of discarding the set.

Once the infusion is completed, the administration set should be discarded. There are two reasons for this recommendation. Blood is an excellent buffer and will neutralize the pH of the intravenous fluid used after the blood transfusion. Also, blood contains protein, which encourages the proliferation of a wide spectrum of organisms.

Microaggregate Blood Filters

The removal of microaggregates can be accomplished by one of two types of microaggregate blood filters. These are classified as either depth or screen filters. Some commonly used microaggregate blood filters are listed in Table 2-1.[7]

Depth filters remove particles by impaction and adsorption. The fluid travels a tortuous path, causing particles in the fluid to be trapped by the filter media and adsorbed. The filter media has many layers in order to create a sufficient number of adsorptive sites. Depth filters do not have an absolute pore size. They have a nominal pore size rating that is determined statistically by challenging the filter with a variety of particles of known size. The Bentley, Fenwal and Swank filters are examples of depth microaggregate filters.

Screen filters operate on a direct interception principle. The filter medium has pores of a predetermined size, thereby intercepting any particle that is larger than the pore size. Screen filters have an

Table 2-1. Characteristics of Currently Available Blood Filters*

Filters	Type	Pore Size (Microns)	Material	Manufacturers Recommended # of Units (Whole Blood)	Priming Volume	Absolute Retention Rate (Diameter of Largest Particle Which Could Still Pass Through Filter)	Contra-indications for Use	Unloading and Channelling of Particles	Contact Area of Blood and Filter Material	Cost Per Filter: Alone-with Set
Microaggregate Blood Filters										
PALL SQ40S	Screen	40 μm	Polyester screen	10 units	20 cc	Retains particles greater than 40 μm	None known	No	Relatively small	$4.80–$7.05
BENTLEY Pff100	Depth	265 μm 60 μm 20 μm	Screen filter (2 layers of polyurethane foam)	5–10 units	80 cc	Cannot be determined	Not for use with fresh blood, platelet & platelet concentrates	Possible	Relatively large	$5.30 (alone)
SWANK 2010	Depth	16 μm to 20 μm	Dacron wool fiber	4–6 units	70 cc	Cannot be determined	Not for use during transfusion of platelet packs of fresh whole blood used as primary therapy for thrombo-cytopenia platelet dysfunction or	Possible	Relatively large	$1.85–$6.40

Table 2-1. Characteristics of Currently Available Blood Filters*—Continued

Filters	Type	Pore Size (Microns)	Material	Manufacturers Recommended # of Units (Whole Blood)	Priming Volume	Absolute Retention Rate (Diameter of Largest Particle Which Could Still Pass Through Filter)	Contraindications for Use	Unloading and Channelling of Particles	Contact Area of Blood and Filter Material	Cost Per Filter: Alone- with Set
FENWAL 4C2423	Depth	20 μm	Nonwoven polyester fibers	5–10 units	60 cc	Cannot be determined	Not for use with fresh blood. Filtration is not advised if specific replacement of platelets and WBCs is desired	Possible	Relatively large	$5.34–$7.47
HEMA™ 9131 or 9132	Combo screen and depth	Over 90 μm 50–90 μm 20 μm	Special proprietary composite (screen depth rolled around screen depth). Removes	2–4 units	60 cc	Cannot be determined	Do not use when transfusing platelet packs, platelet concentrates or platelet-rich plasma	Possible	Relatively large	$5.00–$8.00

similar conditions

Device	Type	Pore Size	Material	Capacity	Volume	Particle Retention	Platelets		Size	Cost*
PEDIATRIC FILTER FENWAL 4C2428	Depth	20 μm	Nonwoven polyester fiber, debris in multiple stages	Up to 10 40 ml aliquots	8–9 cc	No information at this time	Not for use with platelets	No	No information at this time	$4.04–$8.00
Standard Blood Administration Sets										
FENWAL Straight Type Blood Recipient Set 4C2116	Clot screen	170 μm	Lexan plastic nylon mesh	1–2 units	8 cc	Retains particles greater than 170 μm	None stated	Unclear	Relatively small	$2.45–$3.78
FENWAL Double 80-Micron screen Filter Sets 4C2431 or 4C2199	Double screen	200 μm 80 μm	Polyester screen	4 units	30 cc	No information at this time	None stated	No	Relatively small	$2.18–$3.51

*As of June 1984. Used with permission from Schell.[7]

absolute pore size rating. The Pall Ultipor filter, an example of a screen microaggregate filter, has a pore size of 40 microns in diameter.

Microaggregate blood filters are available in administration sets with a number of features available to meet specific needs. They may be single-lead (one bag spike) or multiple-lead filters. Tubing varies, with some manufacturers offering wide-bore tubing for a wider flow range, thereby allowing for a host of patient flow requirements. Sampling sites and in-line coupling ports are also available.

Multiple-lead blood filters are frequently used for blood administration. Normal saline is attached to one coupler, and the venipuncture is then made and maintained while the blood is obtained. The Y-type configuration of the set allows for the sterile transfer of saline into the blood bag for a freer flow during transfusion. In cases of a transfusion reaction, the normal saline is readily available for use while the blood is instantly discontinued.

As a precautionary measure, it is advisable to have the blood filter above the Y-site of the set to ensure that the filter will not be washed out with saline at the end of the transfusion. Washing through the filter could potentially affect retention of debris with some of these filters.[8, 9]

Needle and Catheter Selection

Advances in catheter technology have produced catheters to meet the patient's every need, from the simplest peripheral infusion to the most sophisticated therapy. Infusion may be administered through a catheter or metal needle. There are several types of catheters available on the market.

Types of Catheters

Over-the-Needle Catheter (ONC)

This device is referred to as a plastic needle and is the most commonly used device for blood and fluids. This catheter is inserted in the following fashion: After the venipuncture is made, the catheter is slipped off the needle into the vein. These needles are used to ensure a ready route for the administration of fluid and blood. Their use serves a purpose when there is difficulty keeping the needle in the vein.

These needles can also be converted to heparin locks by inserting a plastic adapter plug onto the needle. Instilling heparin solution

(10–100 units and 1 cc NaCl) or normal saline (0.5 to 1 cc) into the catheter at regular intervals will keep these needles patent for use.

In-the-Needle Catheter (INC)

This catheter is used whenever a longer length catheter is desired for the infusion of drugs or hypertonic solutions, which may cause neurosis if extravasation occurs. This catheter affords less risk of infiltration than the metal needle. It is inserted in the following fashion: After the venipuncture is made, the catheter is pushed through the needle until the desired length is within the wall of the vein. The metal needle is removed from the vein, and its cutting edge is covered by a shield. This prevents catheter severing.

Scalp Vein Needle

This needle is similar to the old metal cannula, which was used for infusion prior to the advent of plastic needles. The metal cannula has been shortened, and the metal hub replaced by two flexible wings. The scalp vein needle was originally designed for use in pediatrics and geriatrics. Today, it can be used in prolonged IV therapy for all ages. It ranges in size from 16- to 23-gauge bore.

There are two types of scalp vein needles available for use. They are:

1. The INT. This device is used for the intermittent administration of fluids or antibiotics. It has a short length of plastic tubing with a resealable injection site. A dilute solution of heparin (usually 10–100 units and 1 cc of NaCl) maintains patency of the needle when not in use.
2. The keep open. This scalp vein needle has a variable length of plastic tubing permanently attached to a female leur adapter, which accommodates an administration set.

Over-the-Wire Catheter

Institutions are now considering the over-the-wire technique for catheter placement. This would avoid shearing of the catheter that could potentially occur during the INC insertion technique. After the venipuncture is made, a guide wire is inserted and the catheter is inserted into the patient over the wire until the desired length is within the lumen of the vein. The needle is removed and only the catheter remains in place, leaving no cutting edge to cover. This procedure is a little more time-consuming and not preferred in the emergency placement situation.

In-lying Catheter

This catheter is used when peripheral access has been exhausted or is not available, such as for patients in shock, obese patients whose veins are obscured, or patients whose access is lost due to prolonged IV therapy. This catheter is inserted by a physician who performs a cutdown on a vein. Once the catheter is threaded into the vein, it is sutured in place.

Insertion of the Cannula

The infusion device is selected based on the purpose of the infusion and the condition and availability of the patient's veins. Red blood cells and whole blood can usually be administered through an 18- or 19-gauge plastic or steel needle. Other blood components may be infused with smaller gauge needles. In patients who have small veins, it may be necessary to use a thin-walled, 23-gauge scalp vein needle. This 23-gauge scalp vein needle is also used, in general, for pediatric transfusion and in adults whose large veins are inaccessible. Long-term catheters are more comfortable if infusions are to continue for a long period of time, and are less likely to cause infiltration complications.

Once a device is chosen, the transfusionist makes certain that the equipment is sterile. Entering a patient's vein is like opening a door to the circulatory system. That is why any IV therapy procedure poses such a great infection risk. Infection can be caused by contaminated equipment, solutions, bacteria transmitted by physical contact, the patient's own bacteria and airborne bacteria. As numerous as these hazards are, they can be prevented or minimized by practicing two simple aseptic techniques consistently:
1. Make sure the equipment is sterile. Take care not to contaminate the equipment during the procedure.
2. Hands should be thoroughly washed for at least 3 minutes, preferably with a hexachlorophene or iodophor preparation, prior to performing any procedure on the patient.

Prior to the venipuncture, the blood administration set is primed with normal saline or blood and cleared of air prior to venipuncture. The tourniquet is placed and the vein is palpated.

Thorough cleansing of the venipuncture site prior to the insertion of the needle or cannula is essential. An aseptic technique is used to prevent the introduction of microorganisms into the patient. Neither aqueous-benzalkonium-like compounds nor hexachlorophene should be used to scrub the IV site. Tincture of iodine (1%–2%) is preferred, but chlorhexidine, iodophors or 70% alcohol can be used.[10] The antiseptic should be applied liberally, starting from the middle and moving in concentric circles outward; the antiseptic is allowed to remain in contact with the skin for at least 30 seconds prior to venipuncture.

The venipuncture is performed using a nontouch technique, and the catheter is advanced into the vein. The tourniquet is released, and the administration set is attached. The infusion is started and the rate adjusted. The site is observed for any signs of infiltration. The catheter is taped to avoid any movement. An accepted topical antibiotic or antiseptic ointment should be applied at the IV site immediately after a successful cannula placement. A sterile dressing should be applied to cover the insertion site. The dressing, and not the tape, should cover the wound, unless the tape is sterile.[10]

The IV tubing is usually looped and taped to the dressing, and the date, time, type and gauge of the catheter and initials of the person who inserted the device are recorded on the dressing. When the saline is properly infusing, attach the administration set to the blood bag by inserting the curved tip connector into a blood bag port. Open the blood slide clamp and gently squeeze and release the bag until the blood flows into the drip chamber. Close the saline clamp. Set the infusion rate at the rate the physician has ordered. Maintaining the drip chamber at ½ full throughout the entire transfusion will enable observation of the fluid flow to the patient. If the entire drip chamber were full, impaired flow would not be easily detected. After the unit of blood has been administered, close the side clamp before air can enter the tubing. If transfusion of other units of blood is to follow, saline may be used to maintain flow between blood units. Hospital policy should state the maximum length of time a catheter should remain in place.

Management of IV Lines

Intravenous needles and catheters are maintained aseptically and changed as often as required. The Centers for Disease Control (CDC) recommends that a peripheral catheter should not be left in place over a 72-hour period, with a 48-hour change preferred. Once the IV needle is in place, the site should be visually checked frequently through the intact dressing. Dressing changes over the catheter site should be done at 48- to 72-hour intervals. If, however, for some reason the dressing becomes unocclusive, a dressing change should be done at that time. The solution administration set should be changed every 48 hours. However, if blood is found in the IV line, the IV administration set should be changed.

Routine collection of blood samples through the IV catheter is not good practice. Blood samples should be taken from other venous sites. In some instances, a patient's venous supply will be exhausted, and the central IV line may be the only access. In these instances, the flow of the IV solution would be shut off, entry made to the catheter only after thorough cleansing of the hub or injection port, and the first 10 cc of blood obtained and discarded. The blood sample can then be obtained.

Whenever there is a transfusion or infusion being administered to a patient, air should never be allowed to enter the transfusion system. However, if air does enter the administration set between transfusions, shut off the flow of fluid to the patient and expel the air from the system. Air is removed by a needle and syringe after cleansing of the entry port.

For optimum maintenance of IV lines, there are a few other recommendations by the CDC[10] that should be observed:
1. Between changes of components, the IV system should be maintained as a closed system as much as possible. All entries into the tubing, as far as administration of medication, should be made through injection ports that are disinfected just before entry.
2. Keep-open solutions, terminated temporarily for drug therapy or blood infusion, must be sterilely capped.
3. Flushing or irrigation of the catheter to improve flow should be avoided. Infusion needles with impaired flow should be replaced.

Rate of Transfusion

The rate of the transfusion is governed by the blood component being infused and the clinical condition of the patient. There is no definite rule for the maximum time a transfusion should take.

When transfusing a unit of blood or RBCs, the transfusion is started at a slow rate for the first 15 minutes to avoid infusion of a large quantity of blood in case of an immediate reaction. In a normal patient, a unit of red cells may be given in 1-½ to 2 hours. Whenever possible, blood should be infused within a 4-hour period. There is a danger of bacterial growth and red cell hemolysis when blood is kept at room temperature for longer periods of time.

Patients who are in danger of fluid overload or in congestive failure require infusions be given over a much longer period of time. In these situations, blood may have to be infused over a 6- to 8-hour interval. When a longer transfusion time is clinically indicated, that information should be communicated to the blood bank. The blood unit may then be divided by the blood bank and the portion of blood not being transfused immediately may be kept in the blood bank under proper refrigeration.

If blood is infusing more slowly than desired, steps to investigate and correct the problem include the following:

1. Elevate the IV pole to increase gravitational pressure
2. Check the patency of the needle
3. Check the flow clamp to be sure it is open
4. Examine the filter of the set for excessive debris; change if necessary
5. As the infusion progresses, red cells tend to settle and slow the infusion; mixing the bag every 30 minutes remedies this problem
6. If red cells are flowing too slowly, add 50 to 100 ml of normal saline to the red cells, provided that the patient can tolerate additional saline.

Calculating Rate of Flow

To calculate the correct flow rate for a patient, it is necessary to determine how much solution the physician ordered and how much time is allowed for the delivery. To calculate the rate of milliliters per hour, the amount of solution to be administered is divided by the delivery time. For example:

$$\frac{1000 \text{ ml}}{8 \text{hr}} = 125 \text{ ml/hr}$$

Next, the type of drip system to be used is decided. If a lot of fluid is being delivered in a short period of time, a macrodrip system is used. Depending upon the manufacturer, the macrodrip takes 10, 15 or 20 drops to deliver 1 ml of fluid. If a small amount of fluid is being delivered over a long period of time, a microdrip system is used. The microdrip takes 60 drops to deliver 1 ml of fluid. The formula to use, then, for either drip system is:

$$\frac{\text{drops/ml}}{60 \text{ min/hr}} \times \frac{\text{amount of fluid/hr}}{1} = \text{drops/min}$$

Once the rate is determined, the flow of the IV is set by timing the number of drops for 1 minute with a watch. The drip rate is adjusted to the rate desired. The rate is periodically checked by using this method. Sudden patient moves or clamp movements may affect the rate. The patient should be reminded not to tamper with the clamp.

Compatible IV Solutions

The transfusion of blood components such as RBCs, platelets or leukocytes may require the use of normal saline (0.9%). AABB *Standards* is very explicit in stating that no medication or intravenous solutions other than normal saline may be added to blood or components prior to or during transfusion.[1(p 31)]

Usually, normal saline is used for dilution of red cells to reduce their viscosity during transfusion, thus allowing for increased flow rates and a decreased hemolysis of the cell. Normal saline, the only acceptable fluid, may also be used in manipulating platelet concentrates for transfusion, or may be used to rinse cryoprecipitate from the bag. Normal saline should also be used to initiate the infusion of whole blood, red cells, leukocytes or platelets.

Hypertonic or hypotonic solutions are completely contraindicated for blood transfusion therapy. Blood components should never be infused with 5% dextrose, as this hypotonic solution causes water to invade the red cells until they burst—resulting in hemolysis. It also causes clumping of red cells in the tubing. Using hypertonic solutions to dilute blood reverses this process and red cells shrink, also resulting in damage.

Lactated Ringer's solution contains enough ionized calcium to overcome the anticoagulant effect of CPD, thus allowing small clots to develop, which then enter the patient's circulation. The effect of 5% dextrose in 0.9 saline and 5% dextrose in 0.4% saline on CPD blood[11,12] apparently shows no more damage to red cells than 0.9% normal saline, and should cause no clinical problems. However, they offer no greater benefits for use than normal saline.

Transfusion Equipment

The use of specialized transfusion devices, such as pressure infusion devices and blood warmers, in certain situations can be lifesaving. However, inappropriate handling of these devices can be detrimental to the recipient.

Pressure Infusion Devices

In certain instances where patients need large amounts of blood rapidly, a blood pump is used. It is recommended that blood pumps only be used with a large-bore needle in place, as flow at high pressure through small-gauge needles may damage red cells. There are two types of pumps that are commonly accepted for use.

The pressure bag is the most commonly used device for increasing flow rates during transfusion. This device has a pump envelope into which the blood bag is inserted. To use the pressure bag, the unit of blood is placed into the pump envelope. One pump envelope loop is slipped through the blood bag loop and the other pump envelope loop is pulled through it. The device is suspended on an

IV pole and the line is connected to the patient. The flow clamp is then opened on the administration set.

The pressure bag is inflated with air by squeezing the pressure bulb. The pressure bulb is squeezed until the desired flow rate is reached. The pressure bag is equipped with a pressure gauge, and the pressure exerted on the unit of blood should never exceed 300 mmHg. Above that level, the pressure may damage the red cells or cause the line to disconnect.

Pressure is exerted evenly on the blood bag using this device. As the blood bag empties, the pressure decreases; therefore, frequent observation of this device is necessary. The pressure bag is reinflated as needed. The flow rate to the patient is checked, and the flow clamp readjusted as necessary. This procedure is repeated with each new unit of blood. Careful observation of the IV site during this procedure is a must. If the vein being used is too small to accept blood under pressure, the blood may infiltrate.

Another type of blood pump used is the built-in blood pump. This blood pump operates with manual pressure, and is built into the blood administration set. It lies below the blood filter of the set.

To use this device, the blood administration set is primed in the usual fashion. The lower pump chamber is inverted and both clamps are opened. The pump chamber and the rest of the IV line are filled and the line is connected to the IV catheter. To administer the blood using this pump, both clamps are opened all the way. Manual pressure is applied by squeezing and releasing the pump chamber. Blood is thus forced down the tubing and into the patient. The pump chamber must be completely refilled before squeezing and releasing it again. This should be continued until the blood bag is nearly empty. To administer the blood without continuing to use the pump, simply stop pumping and adjust the flow rate for a normal straight-line administration.

In the operating room, the most commonly used pump is the Y-type blood pump administration set. The in-line bulb pump in this set is used for alternate pressure administration from the blood bag and the IV solution container. Blood is pumped with this set until the blood bag is nearly empty. The IV solution continues to run after the blood has been administered.

Blood Warmers

Patients receiving one to three units of blood slowly over several hours show no evidence of additional benefit from blood warming. Therefore, blood is not routinely warmed before transfusion. There are, however, some reasonable qualifying situations when warming of blood to body temperature is appropriate. Cold bank blood should be warmed to body temperature when administered in large amounts or when given rapidly, such as in the case of massive hemorrhage. Warming of the blood prevents general body and cardiac hypothermia. In a hypothermic state, the human body is unable to withstand blood loss, and chilling of the myocardium increases the risk of ventricular fibrillation. These two effects of hypothermia may jeopardize the patient's life. Warming of the blood to body temperature decreases these two effects in patients. Warm blood is usually used also in transfusions to patients with potent cold agglutinins, and is usually required in exchange transfusions of newborns.

An effective blood warmer should provide a temperature of above 32 C at flows of 150 ml per minute (one unit of blood in 3 minutes).[13] Conversely, overheating of blood may cause hemolysis, thus the warming device should have an upper limit of 41 C. To ensure safe administration of warm blood, the blood warming system should be equipped with a visible thermometer, and ideally, an audible warning system.

The warming of blood is usually accomplished by using either the waterbath coil or dry-heat warmer. Microwave instruments are available for warming blood, but these warming devices are uneven in their heating and serious hemolysis remains a problem with their use.

Several manufacturing companies[14] have devised units consisting of blood-warming coils that are placed in warm waterbaths. The warming of the blood is accomplished during its passage through the blood coil transfusion set immersed in the waterbath. There are two types of available waterbaths, agitated and nonagitated. The nonagitated water bath is easily used and is the most common type. The straight-line infusion set is primed. The coil is then removed from its sterile wrapper and the clamps are closed. Using aseptic technique, the blood line's male adapter is attached to the coil's female adapter. All clamps are opened and the blood coil is primed. Allow plenty of time for the coil to fill. The clamp nearest the needle is then closed.

The coil is then immersed in a waterbath warmed to 37.6 C. The adapters must stay dry during this procedure or water may enter the tubing, contaminating the entire set. During transfusion, the temperature of the bath must be observed to prevent a pronounced fall in the temperature and thus to the patient. The blood coil is disposable and should be discarded after 24 hours. Extra caution must be taken during use of the waterbath method by placing a thermometer in the water to check the temperature prior to the administration of the blood.

Agitated waterbaths rely upon electrical motors to speed convection and ensure rapid heat transfer to the blood coil. Caution is observed in their use around explosive anesthetics, as sparks from any part of this machinery would be potentially hazardous. These devices should have a nonremovable tag attached to them which will indicate methods of safe operation.

An alternative to the waterbath is the Fenwal Dry-Heat Blood Warmer. The disposable blood warming bag is suspended between two warming plates that warm the bag and blood. Blood is channeled through the tubing in the warming bag and through integral tubing to the recipient. Heat transference is accomplished as blood flows through this channel. The warming bag is intended for one-time patient use. The dry-heat warmer is equipped with a digital temperature display and an audible temperature alarm and shutoff system.

Quality control with warming devices should be a continuing careful procedure. In many hospitals, this responsibility is carried out by the Medical Engineering Department. The safety of the unit, the output temperature and acceptable flow rates are the important areas of concern to be scrutinized during service of these devices.

Other safety measures to be kept in mind when using warm blood for transfusion are fairly standard considerations when dealing with blood transfusion. Blood that cannot be administered to the patient within 30 minutes of receipt from the blood bank should be returned to the blood bank for proper storage. Once blood is warmed, it cannot be returned to the blood bank for reissue.

Neonatal Considerations

The previous discussion has dealt with blood transfusion to the adult. It would seem reasonable to extend the patient protection techniques to neonatal and other pediatric patients.

In neonates, the pulmonary vasculature is still hypertensive and the lumen of vessels is still underdeveloped. Also, the reticuloendothelial system is not fully functional; the lungs, therefore, cannot be cleared of debris. Furthermore, at least 90% of neonates exhibit some type of pulmonary compromise. These considerations suggest the need for microaggregate filtration in the neonate. As with adults, blood components for neonates must be filtered prior to their administration. The protection of microaggregate filtration can now be offered to the neonate as well as the adult.

There is still a great deal of controversy regarding the need for microaggregate filtration for neonates. Some clinicians believe the 170- to 200-micron clot screen is adequate for most neonatal transfusions. Microaggregate filters do have a theoretical role in neonatal transfusion therapy, since microaggregates may accumulate in the pulmonary microcirculation and impair alveolar gas exchange, among other possible insults. However, justification for their routine use is still an issue.[15]

Several microaggregate filters have been designed specifically for use with neonates. One such filter employs 4 cm^2 stainless steel mesh filter media. Several problems have been identified with this filter, however. Schmidt[16] discovered that the use of this filter resulted in posttransfusion hemoglobinemia and hemoglobinuria in several cases involving children. His conclusion was that any filter designed to remove microaggregates should have a significant surface area, and that the 4 cm^2 filter grid found in this filter, which was unnamed in the report, may not be sufficient to prevent clogging and the increase of back pressure.

Longhurst[17] found the Hemo-nate™ (Gesco International) filter unacceptable as a pediatric microaggregate filter because it produced excessive hemolysis and was not able to consistently pass adequate volumes of whole blood or packed RBCs before it occluded.

Therefore, microaggregate filters with larger filtering surfaces appear necessary for use with neonates in order to pass adequate volumes of whole blood or packed RBCs. Microaggregate filters designed for adult patients may be used for blood filtration prior to transfusion in pediatric patients. Depth micropore filters should be avoided for platelet or granulocyte transfusion.[18] A 20-micron depth filter, called the Pediatric Transfusion Filter™ (Fenwal), is now available. The control of the rate and volume of blood transfused is of vital concern when infusing the neonate patient. The system used to infuse blood products should be reviewed and a policy established within each institution.

The volume of a transfusion can be measured using a Hemoset with a Cair Clamp, which is a blood infusion set with an in-line burette device (Abbott Laboratories). Microbore extension tubing can be used with prefiltered blood components. Platelet infusion sets offer the shortest tubing available for IV push injections. These sets can be adapted for filtering blood components into a syringe. The component bag is entered using the spiked end of the platelet infusion set. A three-way stopcock is attached to the needle catheter adapter and a syringe is attached. Blood components are then drawn through the filter and into the syringe.

In general, the flow rate for neonatal transfusion is less than 10 ml per hour.[19] Infusion devices could be used to monitor and control the volume and rate of transfusion. Infusion syringes and infusion pumps must be tested to determine whether the flow rate is correct and whether hemolysis has occurred. Warming of blood to room temperature is usually all that is needed prior to the transfusion of blood components. Normal saline can be used to dilute or flush RBCs through the tubing for maximum infusion and the conservation of the blood component.

Conclusion

Blood transfusion is a very complex procedure and can involve a certain amount of risk for the patient. Responsibility for administering this vital fluid increases with the rapid advancement in transfusion therapy. In many hospitals, the registered nurse has become the primary responsible transfusion therapist. However, whether blood is being administered by a physician or a registered nurse, only those individuals trained in every phase of transfusion therapy should hold this responsibility. A thorough knowledge of transfusion devices is critical for the proper administration of blood and blood components.

References

1. Schmidt PJ, ed. Standards for blood banks and transfusion services. 11th ed. Arlington, VA: American Association of Blood Banks, 1984:30.
2. Gianino N. Equipment used for transfusion. In: Rutman RC, Miller WV, eds. Transfusion therapy principles and practices. Rockville, MD: Aspen Systems, 1982:155.
3. Swank RL. Alteration of blood on storage: Measurement of adhesiveness of 'aging' platelets and leukocytes and their removal by filtration. N Engl J Med 1970;265:728–33.
4. McNamara JS, Molot MD, Stremple JF. Screen filtration pressure in combat casualties. Ann Surg 1970;172:334–41.
5. Moseley RV, Doty DB. Changes in the filtration characteristics of stored blood. Ann Thorac Surg 1970;171:329–35.
6. Zeller JA. An electron microscopic study of microaggregates in ACD stored blood. 3rd Congress on Thrombosis and Hemostasis. 1972:264.
7. Schell RD. Blood microfiltration application reviewed. Intravenous Therapy News 1984;11:9.
8. Wenz B. Microaggregate blood filtration and the febrile transfusion reaction. Transfusion 1983;23:95.
9. Eckert G. Prevention of pulmonary microembolism during blood transfusion by means of fine mesh filters. Anästh Intensivther Notfallmed 1980;15:201–6.

10. Simmons BP, Hooten TM, et al. Guidelines for prevention of intravascular infections. NITA 1982;5:39–46.
11. Ryden SE. Compatibility of blood with intravenous solutions. In: Marnette BL, Brzica SM, eds. From vein to vein: A seminar for phlebotomists and transfusionists. Washington, DC: American Association of Blood Banks, 1976:33–6.
12. Ryden SE, Oberman HA. Compatibility of common intravenous solutions with CPD blood. Transfusion 1975;15:250–5.
13. Russell WJ. A review of blood warmers for massive transfusion. Anesthesia and Intensive Care 1974;2:109–30.
14. Webb JW. Contemporary comments on infusion pumps. NITA 1981;4:9–14.
15. Wallas CH. Considerations and indications for the use of red blood cell products. In: Luban N, ed. Hemotherapy of the infant and premature. Arlington, VA: American Association of Blood Banks, 1983:29.
16. Schmidt WF, et al. RBC destruction caused by a micropore blood filter. JAMA 1982;248:1629.
17. Longhurst WM, et al. In vitro evaluation of a pediatric microaggregate blood filter. Transfusion 1983;23:170.
18. Sills RH, et al. Platelet transfusion in the newborn. In: Sherwood WC, et al, eds. Transfusion therapy: The fetus, infant, and child. New York: Masson Publishing, 1980:95–111.
19. Widmann FK, ed. Technical manual. 8th ed. Washington, DC: American Association of Blood Banks, 1981:301.

In: Reynolds, AW and Steckler, D, eds.
Practical Aspects of Blood Administration
Arlington, VA: American Association
of Blood Banks, 1986

3

The Infusion of Blood and Blood Components

Loni Calhoun, MT(ASCP)SBB

*I*NTRAVENOUS (IV) THERAPISTS ARE often more knowledgeable about patient care and infusion equipment than they are about the blood components they infuse. They rely on the expertise of the physician and the blood bank staff to ensure that the product is appropriate, and to provide guidelines for proper administration. However, to maximize the effectiveness and safety of the procedure, the infusionist should keep in mind the following:

1. Why is the product being given?
2. What is in the product?
3. How is it handled and stored?
4. Is it ABO- and Rh-compatible?
5. How should it be administered?
6. What adverse reactions may develop?

Many fine publications already address these topics.[1-4] Blood banks and nursing services are encouraged to make such resources available to their transfusion staff. This chapter will briefly review blood collection and processing with respect to product safety and viability, and then will summarize the six points listed above for the common blood components and derivatives used today.

Blood Collection and Processing

Whole blood is collected from healthy donors who are prescreened with both a medical history and a limited physical exam. Standard acceptability guidelines have been established to protect the donor's health as well as the recipient's.[3] The venipuncture is performed aseptically, with minimum trauma; a good flow rate ensures maximum coagulation factors in the final product. Up to 450 ml blood

Loni Calhoun, MT(ASCP)SBB, Education Coordinator, Blood Bank, UCLA
Medical Center, Los Angeles, California

are collected from the donor into an FDA-approved container with a premeasured amount of anticoagulant.

Several anticoagulant-preservative solutions are licensed for whole blood collection: acid citrate dextrose (ACD), citrate phosphate dextrose (CPD) and CPD adenine-1 (CPDA-1). Their purpose, besides preventing coagulation, is to preserve the life and function of red blood cells. Function relates to a cell's ability to deliver oxygen to the tissues through the generation of 2,3-diphosphoglycerate (2,3-DPG). Viability correlates with the level of adenosine triphosphate (ATP), which is manufactured by the red cells through glycolysis. The maximum length of storage is determined by a viability standard that all solutions must meet: 70% of the transfused red cells must be found in circulation 24 hours after transfusion.[4]

Red cells stored with CPDA-1 meet this requirement up to 35 days. CPDA-1 contains sodium citrate to bind ionized calcium and prevent coagulation, dextrose to support glycolysis for ATP production, citric acid and phosphate to buffer the solution to a pH that balances the preservation of 2,3-DPG and ATP, and adenine, which along with phosphate enhances ATP production.[5] CPDA-1 is the preservative most commonly used today. ACD and CPD are only approved for 21-day storage. Heparin, an approved but rarely used anticoagulant, has a storage limit of 48 hours because it contains no preservatives. It is licensed for red cell components only.

To extend red cell storage to 42 days, additive systems are also available. Whole blood is collected into a primary bag containing CPD or CP2D (CPD with twice the dextrose). After most of the plasma is removed, adenine-saline (AS), a nutritive solution in an attached satellite bag, is added to the packed red cells. The chemical make-up of currently licensed additive systems is compared to CPDA-1 in Table 3-1. Additive systems provide red cells with better viability and permit collection of more plasma for component production.[4]

A unit of blood may be kept as whole blood or may be separated into its component parts: red cells, platelets and plasma. This is accomplished using differential centrifugation and a collection bag with satellites attached by integral tubing (Fig 3-1). The advantages of component separation are twofold. Not all components have the same storage requirements; separation permits each one to be stored for maximum preservation. Component production also allows several patients to benefit from one donation, thereby conserving a valuable resource.

At the time of donation, additional samples of donor blood are collected and tested for ABO, Rh and unexpected antibodies. The serum must also test negative for hepatitis B surface antigen, syphilis

Table 3-1. Comparison of CPDA-1 and Currently Licensed Additive Systems

Chemical	CPDA-1 (g/63 ml)	Adsol® System*		Nutricel® System**	
		Primary Bag CPD (g/63 ml)	Additive AS-1 (g/100 ml)	Primary Bag CP2D (g/63 ml)	Additive AS-3 (g/100 ml)
Sodium Citrate	1.66	1.66	—	1.66	0.588
Dextrose	2.01	1.61	2.2	3.22	1.10
Citric Acid	0.206	0.206	—	0.206	0.042
NaH₂PO₄	0.140	0.140	—	0.140	0.276
Adenine	0.017	—	0.027	—	0.030
Mannitol	—	—	0.750	—	—
Sodium Chloride	—	—	0.900	—	0.410

* Fenwal Laboratories
**Cutter Biological

and HTLV-III antibody before it can be used. Test results are indicated on the blood container label. If blood must be used for an emergency before testing is complete, the label will conspicuously indicate this fact and testing will be completed as soon as possible.

Other landmarks on the unit label that an infusionist must be familiar with are the name of the product, its unique donor number, the expiration date and, if appropriate, expiration time, and a reference to a circular of information on the use of blood (available from the collecting facility and equivalent to a drug package insert). Statements of caution are also given. Although careful donor screening and laboratory tests help ensure the safety of the blood

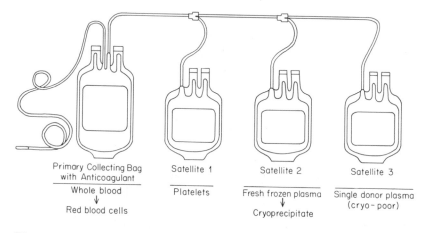

Primary Collecting Bag with Anticoagulant	Satellite 1	Satellite 2	Satellite 3
Whole blood ↓ Red blood cells	Platelets	Fresh frozen plasma ↓ Cryoprecipitate	Single donor plasma (cryo-poor)

Figure 3-1. A quadruple blood bag set and the blood components routinely prepared from it.

supply, blood components may still transmit disease. Federal law prohibits dispensing them without a physician's prescription.

Red Blood Cell Components

Red cell transfusions are given to patients who have become symptomatic from an oxygen-carrying capacity deficit. This may develop from blood loss, bone marrow failure or shortened red cell survival. A number of components are available for transfusion; each has special characteristics and indications. Good clinical evaluation is needed before transfusion is started to assess the cause and extent of the deficiency and to determine the best course of action. Transfusions should not be performed when the problem can more effectively and safely be managed with medications or simple surgical intervention. In a stable patient, one unit of red cells will increase the hemoglobin 1 g/dl and the hematocrit 3%.[4] In infants, 3 ml red cells/kg body weight will increase the hemoglobin 1 g/dl.[6]

Whole Blood

A unit of whole blood contains the red cell and plasma elements of donor blood plus the anticoagulant. Its total volume is approximately 515 ml with a hematocrit of 36-40%.[2] The supply of whole blood is limited because most units are used in the preparation of components. Depending on community demand and manufacturing schedules, blood centers may prepare modified whole blood. Platelets and/or cryoprecipitate can be removed from freshly collected donor units and the remaining plasma returned to the original bag to "reconstitute" the red cells to whole blood. Modified whole blood is used interchangeably with stored whole blood; however, it may have 30–40% less fibrinogen if cryoprecipitate was harvested.[4]

Blood stored more than 24 hours at 1–6 C has few viable platelets and granulocytes. These cells degenerate and, along with fibrin strands, make up the microaggregates seen in blood stored more than a few days.[7] Viable lymphocytes persist through the entire storage period. Heat labile coagulation Factors V and VIII decrease, but levels of 30% Factor V and 15–20% Factor VIII have been reported in whole blood stored 21 days.[8,9] These levels are not sufficient to correct specific factor deficiencies in bleeding patients. Stable coagulation Factors II, VII, IX, X and fibrinogen are well-maintained throughout the storage period.

Biochemical changes also take place in blood during storage at 1–6 C (see Table 3-2). Sugar levels and pH drop as red cells undergo anaerobic glycolysis to generate ATP; the end product of this met-

Table 3-2. Biochemical Changes in Whole Blood Stored in CPDA-1 for 35 Days[2]

	Storage (Days)		
	0	35	Reference
Plasma Dextrose (mg/dl)	432	282	10
Whole Blood Lactate (mg/dl)	19	202	10
Whole Blood pH	7.16	6.73	10
Red Cell 2,3-DPG (μMol/gHb)	13.2	0.7	11
Red Cell ATP (μMol/gHb)	4.18	2.40	11
Plasma Potassium (mEq/l)	3.3	17.2	10
Plasma Sodium (mEq/l)	169	153	10
Whole Blood Ammonia (μg/dl)	82	703	10

abolic pathway is lactic acid. The drop in pH decreases 2,3-DPG and the cell's ability to release oxygen to the tissues. As metabolic functions slow in the cold temperature, ATP levels decrease. Red cells no longer regulate the sodium-potassium gradient across their membranes as efficiently and plasma potassium increases. Ammonia levels also increase.

These storage changes have little significance in most transfusion situations; patients compensate for or reverse them. Up to 50% 2,3-DPG can be regenerated within 3–8 hours after transfusion.[12] However, severely compromised patients and the very young do not tolerate these changes, especially in 2,3-DPG. Therefore, blood less than 7 days old is recommended for neonatal transfusion.[4]

Whole blood is the product of choice when both volume replacement and oxygen-carrying capacity are needed, eg, for exchange transfusions and for actively bleeding patients in hemorrhagic shock. When volume can no longer be sustained with crystalloid solutions alone, and colloids become necessary (a blood loss of one third the blood volume or more), whole blood is preferred.[4] It is a safer and less expensive therapy than using both red cells and plasma. Whole blood should not be used when volume overload is a concern.

Red Blood Cells

A unit of red cells, also called packed red cells, is prepared by removing 200–250 ml of plasma from a whole blood unit after centrifugation or sedimentation. It has a volume of approximately 300 ml with a hematocrit not exceeding 80%. Some residual plasma is left with the red cells to ensure their preservation during storage. Red cells prepared with additive solutions have less plasma, but the nutrient solution gives them a greater total volume, approximately 350 ml, and a hematocrit of 55–65%.[1] It also gives them increased sugar/mannitol concentrations. Mannitol can produce diuresis, but the level in an AS-1 unit is much less than the 1–2 g/kg body weight dose needed for this effect.[1] If mannitol or sugar levels become a concern in massive transfusion situations, the solution can be removed before transfusion.

Red cells are the component of choice for patients with chronic anemia, liver, cardiac or kidney disease, and patients who cannot tolerate rapid changes in blood volume. The reduced plasma volume eliminates unwanted plasma chemicals and decreases the risk of circulatory overload. Red cells are also used for routine blood loss in surgery. Small losses of 1000 ml or less can be replaced with crystalloid/colloid solutions alone. However, when oxygen-carrying capacity is needed, as it may be in up to 65% of surgeries,[13] red blood cells are appropriate. If significant volume expansion is also needed, whole blood is preferred, but red cells and volume expanders may be substituted if whole blood is not available.

Leukocyte-Poor Red Blood Cells

Red cells may be modified by centrifugation, washing, filtration or a combination of these techniques to make them leukocyte-poor. By definition, 70% of the leukocytes have been removed and at least 70% of the red cells have been retained. The final volume of the product and the efficiency of leukocyte removal varies with the method of preparation.[14] Saline wash methods are commonly used to prepare leukocyte-poor red cells, but such products are expensive and expire 24 hours from the time of preparation. Recently, microaggregate filtration of centrifuged red cells has been found to effectively remove leukocytes.[15,16] This method is cost-effective and does not shorten the expiration date before transfusion.

Leukocyte-poor red blood cells are indicated for patients experiencing repeated febrile nonhemolytic reactions to blood transfusion. Patients with a history of multiple pregnancies and/or transfusions may develop antibodies to leukocytes and/or platelets. These may react with the white cell and platelet material normally present in red cell components and cause febrile symptoms lasting up to 8 hours. Because patients experiencing one reaction seldom have another with their next transfusion,[17] many transfusion services recommend that leukocyte-poor red cells be given only after two or more such reactions are documented.[4]

Washed Red Blood Cells

Red cells can be washed with normal saline to remove most plasma and non-red-cell elements, plus microaggregates. The final product varies: some red cell mass is lost and remaining cells may be resuspended in saline, with or without dextrose, to a hematocrit of 65–85%.[1] The amount of plasma, leukocyte and platelet contamination also varies with the method and volume of wash solution.

As discussed above, washed red cells may be prepared leukocyte-poor to reduce febrile reactions. They may also be of benefit to patients with a history of severe allergic reactions: generalized urticaria, asthma or anaphylaxis. These reactions are thought to be related to an IgE or IgG reaction to allergens or proteins in the donor plasma. Some patients with anti-IgA may tolerate washed red cells; however, severely sensitized individuals may require components washed with five volumes of saline, frozen-deglycerolized red cells, or products from special IgA-deficient donors.[18] Washed red cells are also requested for patients with paroxysmal nocturnal hemoglobinuria (PNH). Many physicians prefer washed cells to avoid transfusing additional complement and to avoid potential antibody-antigen reactions from transfused leukocytes or plasma which might activate the complement cascade.[19] The need for this more expensive product has been questioned: one group reports no difference in minor febrile reactions between washed red cells versus whole blood and packed red cells in their PNH transfusions.[20]

Deglycerolized Red Blood Cells

To extend storage to 3 years or more, red cells can be frozen after glycerol, a cryoprotective agent, is added. Glycerol enters the cell and prevents damage due to cell dehydration and mechanical injury from ice formation.[21] Two methods are commonly used today: a high-glycerol (40% wt/vol) slow freeze method with storage at −65 C maximum (mechanical freezing) and a low-glycerol (18% wt/vol) rapid freeze method with storage at −120 C (liquid nitrogen).[4] Before transfusion, the glycerol is removed by washing to prevent osmotic hemolysis in vivo. Accepted standards require that methods produce 80% red cell yield postthaw and 70% survival posttransfusion.[3] Units are usually frozen within 6 days of collection to ensure optimal 2,3-DPG and ATP levels after the thaw/deglycerolization process.

Frozen storage is ideal for the long-term preservation of rare and/or autologous donor units. Because the extensive washing required to remove the glycerol also removes leukocytes, platelets and plasma, deglycerolized red cells are suitable for patients with antibodies to these fractions. However, the expense, preparation time, and 24-hour expiration do not make this product practical for the prophylactic prevention of febrile/allergic transfusion reactions or routine inventory control. At one time, deglycerolized red cells were used to prevent alloimmunization in kidney transplant candidates. Data now suggest that cadaver grafts have better survival when whole blood or red cells are used.[22]

Storage and Handling

All red cell components, with the exception of frozen cells, must be stored at 1–6 C in special refrigerators. Fans circulate the air and ensure an even temperature throughout, recorders continuously monitor temperature, and audible alarms alert the staff when temperatures are outside the recommended limits.[3] Storage at 1–6 C slows metabolic functions so that red cells meet viability requirements throughout their approved storage time. It also retards the growth of any bacteria present. During transport from the blood bank to the bedside, blood temperature limits are 1–10 C. At 25 C ambient temperature, the maximum limit is reached in 30 minutes.[23] If the transfusion cannot be started immediately, most transfusion services require that blood components be returned within 30 minutes for proper storage. Components are accepted for reissue only if the blood container closure has not been disturbed.

The approved maximum storage time of the anticoagulant gives a red cell component its expiration date and time: midnight, 21 days after collection for ACD and CPD; 35 days for CPDA-1; 42 days for adenine-saline additives. When a red cell bag is entered to process or modify the product, it is considered potentially contaminated and its expiration changes to 24 hours. The new time and date are clearly indicated on the label. Expiration times apply to blood storage, not transfusion, eg, a unit expiring at midnight may be issued for transfusion 1 minute before midnight and transfused over the next 2–4 hours without concern.

Some blood components require additional handling after they arrive from the donor center. This is preferentially done just before transfusion to avoid prolonged storage of potentially contaminated units. To remove the plasma from a unit of whole blood and make the necessary record changes takes 10 minutes. Saline washing may take 20–30 minutes. Frozen red cells take approximately 15 minutes to thaw and another 45 minutes to deglycerolize. The infusionist must keep these preparation times in mind when ordering blood components. Good communication with the blood bank is needed if the component must be ready at a specific time.

ABO and Rh Compatibility

To appreciate the importance of ABO compatibility in transfusion, the infusionist must understand what compatibility means. The four major blood groups in the ABO system are A, B, AB and O. The letter designation represents the presence of the A or B antigen on the red blood cell. Group A's have only A antigen; group AB's have both A and B; group O has neither. Because the antigen is ubiquitous in nature, infants 3–6 months old develop antibody to the A or B antigen they lack. Hence, group A's make anti-B; group O's make both anti-A and anti-B; group AB's make neither. These antibodies cause the immediate acute hemolytic transfusion reactions seen with ABO-incompatible blood transfusions.

A simple rule to remember when evaluating ABO compatibility between the donor and recipient is this: Never give the patient an antigen or antibody he or she does not already have.[24] Because whole blood contains both red cells and plasma, it must be given as ABO identical. When plasma is removed in the production of red cells and washed or deglycerolized cells, there is more choice in what can be safely given without violating the compatibility rule. A group A recipient may receive either group A or group O red cells. Appendix 3-1 summarizes ABO compatibility.

The Rh or D factor is the second most important antigen to match in transfusion. Rh-positive individuals have the D antigen on their red cells; Rh-negative individuals lack the D antigen. Rh-positive recipients can receive Rh-positive or Rh-negative red cells, but Rh-negative recipients should only receive Rh-negative, because they may make anti-D after exposure to Rh-positive red cells through transfusion or pregnancy. Rarely, Rh-negative patients must be given Rh-positive blood when Rh-negative blood is not available and transfusion needs are urgent. This action is not taken without physician notification and approval.

Tests to detect serological incompatibility must be performed prior to all red cell transfusions. The donor's ABO group is repeated, and Rh type if Rh-negative, to verify the blood label accuracy. The recipient sample is tested for ABO, Rh and significant unexpected antibodies, and the results are checked against past historical records. Donor cells are also tested against patient serum (major crossmatch). If the recipient has been pregnant or transfused within the past 3 months, or if this information is uncertain, the sample used in testing must be collected within 2 days of the transfusion to allow detection of antibodies forming from this potential sensitization.[3] Pretransfusion testing may take 15 minutes to 1 hour, depending on the methods used. An infusionist must be aware of the protocols in the institution because this time is added onto the preparation time of all red cell components. If a significant antibody is detected during pretransfusion testing, it is identified and blood negative for that specific antigen is crossmatched. These additional steps take even more time.

When transfusion is urgently needed before the completion of tests, the patient's physician may sign an "emergency release request" to acknowledge an understanding of the risk involved and an acceptance of responsibility. These forms are available in all transfusion services. The blood bank will complete testing as quickly as possible and will notify the physician of any problems detected. If blood must be transfused before the patient's ABO-Rh is known, group O Rh-negative red blood cells are selected. Once the patient's type is known, ABO-Rh identical units are preferred.

Administration

A discussion of transfusion equipment and its use is presented in Chapter 2. All blood components must be transfused through a filter. This is accomplished by using standard blood infusion sets with in-line filters and drip chambers. Standard filters have a pore size of 170–220 μ; microaggregate filters have pore sizes of 20–40 μ. While either may be used, the microaggregate filter costs more and has few proven indications.[7] Microaggregate filters are not needed for very fresh blood and washed or deglycerolized red cells because these components are relatively "clean." When transfusing a red cell unit that requires microfiltration to render it leukocyte-poor, microaggregate filters must be used. Such units will carry this caution and the transfusion service may supply the special filter.

An 18-gauge needle or catheter is recommended for routine blood transfusion; it is large enough for good flow, but not too big for most veins.[4] Smaller sizes (eg, 23 gauge) may be used for infants and small veins, but they add resistance to the flow rate. Whether they also contribute to hemolysis is unclear.[25] One group of investigators has recently concluded that specific guidelines regulating needle size do not appear justified.[26]

Most transfusions are completed within 2 hours. A slow flow rate should be used at the start, while the patient is closely monitored for signs of acute reaction. Then the rate is increased to complete the transfusion within a reasonable time. Blood should be given as quickly as possible with infusion rates based on the patient's blood volume, cardiac status and hemodynamic condition.[4] Adults tolerate rates up to 1.5 ml/kg/min, although some drop in ionized calcium may be noted at this rate.[27] Infants with cardiac decompression may only tolerate rates of 5 ml/kg/hr.[6]

The maximum time a transfusion may take is not supported by clinical data. Many institutions select 4 hours as a guideline because of the potential risks of contamination.[4] If a patient tolerates only very slow infusion rates, red cells should be used in place of whole blood. Units may also be split into smaller aliquots and each aliquot given over 4 hours. Unused portions can be properly stored in the blood bank until they are needed.

Red cells with high hematocrits may flow more slowly than desired, especially if a small needle is used. To increase the flow rate, 50–100 ml normal saline may be added to the unit, provided the patient is not sodium- or volume-restricted. This is easily accomplished when Y-type infusion sets are used. Whole blood, modified whole blood, washed or deglycerolized red cells, and red cells with additive solutions should not need saline dilution. If slow flow rates are a problem with these components, a more careful investigation of the needle and filter is needed.[28]

Reactions

Recipients can experience a number of adverse reactions during red cell transfusions, some troublesome but insignificant, others life-threatening.[4] The more common problems are classified as febrile nonhemolytic, antibodies in the recipient reacting to donor leukocytes and/or platelets; allergic, recipient antibodies reacting with allergens in the donor plasma; and circulatory overload, giving too much blood too quickly. Hemolytic reactions result from red cell incompatibilities and can be life-threatening. Less common, but equally serious problems include anaphylactic reactions (anti-IgA in the patient reacting with IgA protein in donor plasma) and bacterial contamination in the donor unit.

The symptoms from transfusion reactions are numerous: fever, chills, dyspnea, chest/back pain, headache, nausea, diarrhea, urticaria, wheezing, coughing, cyanosis, pulmonary edema, hemoglobinuria, diffuse bleeding, renal failure and shock. Because symptoms do not confirm the cause, and treatment and prevention vary with the cause, all adverse reactions must be evaluated by the blood bank. Chapter 4 presents a complete discussion of transfusion reactions and appropriate nursing and laboratory responses.

Patients receiving leukocyte-poor, washed or deglycerolized red cells may experience fewer febrile, allergic and anaphylactic reactions. However, *all* red cell components may cause hemolytic reactions, sensitize a patient to alloantigens, initiate graft-versus-host disease (GVHD) in immunocompromised patients or transmit disease, including hepatitis and acquired immune deficiency syndrome (AIDS). Deglycerolized red cells may reduce the risk of cytomegalovirus (CMV) transmission.[29]

Platelets

Platelet transfusions are used to treat surgical and medical patients with active thrombocytopenic bleeding or to prevent bleeding in thrombocytopenic patients. Predicting who will bleed, especially during surgery, is not easy, but platelet counts and Template Bleeding Times may help. Normal platelet counts are 150,000–400,000/mm³. Most surgeries can be safely completed with platelet counts of 60,000–70,000/mm³.[4] Patients with counts of 50,000/mm³ and a bleeding time less than two times the upper limit of normal usually do not need prophylactic platelet transfusions before surgery.[30,31] If thrombocytopenic bleeding develops in surgery, transfusions to restore the count to 70,000/mm³ are necessary. These guidelines also apply in massive transfusion settings, where infusion of 15–20 units of blood may significantly dilute platelet counts below hemostatic levels.[9]

Blood loss from thrombocytopenic hemorrhage is not rapid and usually does not have serious consequences unless it is critically located, eg, the eye.[30] Platelet transfusions are best withheld until rapid bleeding is surgically controlled, or in the case of cardiopulmonary bypass surgery, after the patient is disconnected from the pump. Surgical patients with normal platelet counts but abnormal function, sometimes associated with myeloproliferative and qualitative inherited disorders, might follow the above guidelines.[31]

Prophylactic platelet transfusions are given to nonbleeding patients with rapidly dropping counts or counts below 10,000–20,000/mm³ secondary to cancer, chemotherapy or aplastic disorders.[30] Significant spontaneous bleeds with platelet counts above 20,000/mm³ are rare. Even with counts of 5000–10,000/mm³, only a slight increase in minor bleeding was noted in one group of aplastic patients.[32] The level at which prophylactic platelet transfusions are needed must depend on the physician's clinical assessment and complicating risk factors such as fever, infection and drugs. Because the half-life of platelets is 3–4 days, transfusions may be repeated every 1–3 days until the patient stabilizes or recovers bone marrow function.[1]

Unless there is a serious hemorrhage, platelet transfusions are not helpful in treating thrombocytopenia caused by idiopathic thrombocytopenic purpura (ITP), thrombotic thrombocytopenic purpura (TTP), immune-mediated drug purpura and hypersplenism.[33] The factors responsible for the excessive destruction or sequestration of platelets in these conditions affect all platelets including those transfused. Platelet transfusions will not correct problems from posttransfusion purpura or neonatal isoimmune thrombocytopenic purpura unless Pl^A1 antigen-negative platelets are available or exchange transfusion is attempted in the neonate's case. Platelet dysfunctions caused by extrinsic factors in dysproteinemia and uremia are better managed by plasmapheresis and dialysis respectively.[33] Finally, although platelet transfusions are given in disseminated intravascular coagulapathies (DIC), fibrinogen breakdown products interfere with platelet adhesion and aggregation, which makes transfusion less effective.[34]

Random Donor Platelets

Random donor platelets, known also as platelet concentrates or, simply, platelets, are prepared from units of whole blood within 6 hours of collection. Although standards require that a minimum of 5.5×10^{10} platelets be present in 75% of units tested, many units have much higher counts ($6-8 \times 10^{10}$).[35] These platelets are suspended in enough donor plasma to maintain the pH within the container above 6.0. The plasma volume varies with the method of preparation and intended temperature of storage: 20–30 ml for products stored at 1–6 C and 40–70 ml for products stored at 20–24 C. This plasma contains hemostatic levels of all coagulation factors, which may benefit patients needing both platelets and factor replacement. Factor VIII activity of 68% and Factor V activity of 47% have been reported after 72 hours storage at 22 C.[36] Platelets also contain a significant number of leukocytes (approximately 3×10^8)[35] and small amounts of red cells (trace to 0.5 ml).[4]

One unit of platelets should raise the platelet count 5000–10,000/mm[3] in an average adult and 75,000–100,000/mm[3] in a newborn.[4] This is known as the platelet increment. To assess a transfusion's effectiveness, platelet counts may be checked at 1 hour and 24 hours posttransfusion to determine the increment survival: 60% of the platelets should be circulating after 1 hour and 40% after 24 hours.[30] These increases or survivals will not be observed if fever, infection, splenomegaly or active bleeding are present. Poor recovery in the absence of these factors indicates the patient may be refractory to random donor platelets. Appropriate platelet doses may be calculated using pretransfusion counts, posttransfusion count desired, and the platelet increment. Doses of 1 unit/10 kg body weight have also been recommended for hemostasis[37] and simplify calculations.

Single Donor Platelets

Single donor platelets, also known as plateletpheresis products, are collected by manual or automated methods that return all unneeded portions of the donor's blood back to the donor. One unit contains $3–6 \times 10^{11}$ platelets suspended in 200–400 ml fresh donor plasma. Depending on the method of collection, this product may also be significantly contaminated with leukocytes ($0.03–6 \times 10^9$) and red cells (trace to 20 ml).[38] A single donor platelet is equivalent to 6–8 units of random donor platelets and will raise the average adult platelet count 30,000–60,000/mm³.[4]

Single donor platelets are the ideal product for treating patients who have developed HLA antibodies from previous transfusions and have become refractory or unresponsive to random donor platelets.[39] Because red cells are returned to the donor in the collection process, apheresis donors may give the equivalent of 6–8 units of random platelets several times a week.[3] This permits efficient use of special HLA-matched or designated donors. Using HLA-matched donors to prevent HLA alloimmunization is controversial.[30] Unmatched single donor platelets are sometimes given to nonrefractory patients when platelet inventories are low; however, this is not recommended because they are more expensive to prepare, make greater demands on the donor and may have a shorter shelf life. People who have ingested aspirin within the past 3 days should not be used as the single source of platelets[2] because aspirin interferes with platelet function.

Storage and Handling

Shelf life for platelets depends on a complex combination of factors: platelet count, plasma volume, pH, temperature, container and agitation.[40] Platelets are either stored at 1–6 C with no agitation and expire in 48 hours, or they are stored at 20–24 C with continuous agitation and expire in 72 hours or 5 days, depending on the plastic formulation of the storage bag.[4] Data show that platelets stored 20–24 C have superior function and viability[41] and these are the products routinely supplied today. "Room temperature" platelets must not be refrigerated. Single donor platelets are also stored at 20–24 C with continuous agitation and expire in 24 hours or 5 days, depending on the method of collection and storage bag.

Platelets can be transfused with no further preparation; however, to simplify their infusion, many blood banks pool units of random donor platelets into one bag. Once the sterility of a bag is broken, products stored at room temperature expire in 6 hours.[3] Pooling many bags together increases the risk of contamination and FDA recommends an expiration of 4 hours for pooled platelets. Either special platelet pooling sets with multiple leads or transfer bags with a single lead may be used. The pooling process adds 15–30 minutes preparation time to the request.

Patients who cannot tolerate the plasma volume of pooled platelets or ABO plasma incompatibilities may be given volume-reduced platelets. Platelets are centrifuged (6–20 minutes), then are allowed to "dissociate" or "resuspend" for 20–80 minutes.[42] Preparation must start well in advance of the transfusion.

Platelets may also be made leukocyte-poor to reduce the incidence of febrile nonhemolytic reactions and to increase platelet recovery in alloimmunized patients. Single donor platelets can be prepared as leukocyte-poor during the collection process. Random donor platelets are made leukocyte-poor after collection by centrifugation[4] or filtration. This is not a routine procedure in most transfusion services and should be ordered in advance. The process adds an additional 15–30 minutes to the preparation time. Centrifugation removes 85–95% of the leukocytes and 20–30% of the platelets.[43,44] Filtration with Terumo® microaggregate filters removes 90% of the leukocytes and 7.5% of the platelets[44]; the author's laboratory finds 90–95% leukocyte removal.

Washing platelets with non-plasma solutions may benefit patients who have severe reactions to pooled or volume-reduced platelets. This procedure may take more than 1 hour to complete and the product should be transfused within 1 hour of preparation.[45] Frozen storage of platelets at −80 C is possible with the cryoprotective agent dimethylsulfoxide (DMSO).[21,33] This research technology produces 40–70% platelet recovery and may be indicated for the extended storage (3 years) of autologous platelets from refractory donors who are not currently thrombocytopenic. To thaw the product and remove DMSO prior to infusion may also take more than 1 hour.

ABO and Rh Compatibility

Although it is ideal to give platelets as ABO identical, few blood banks have the inventory to support this practice. ABO antigen is present on the platelet membrane. Some studies report a slight decrease in recovery of ABO-incompatible platelets over ABO-compatible; others report no change.[30,33] Another concern is the amount of A or B antibody in the plasma and its potential to hemolyze recipient red cells. AABB *Standards* recommends that platelet plasma be ABO-compatible with the patient's red cells, especially when transfusing neonates.[3] Selection choices are summarized in Appendix 3-1. Because prompt transfusion is more important to patient therapy than waiting for compatible platelet products, patients may be given any ABO type.

There is no D antigen on platelet membrane.[33] However, Rh-negative recipients are at small risk of becoming sensitized to D by red cells present in Rh-positive platelet products: only 8% of immunosuppressed Rh-negative patients receiving 80–110 Rh-positive units developed anti-D in one study.[46] For this reason, Rh-negative platelets are preferred for Rh-negative females who may bear children. If this group must receive Rh-positive platelets, the physician may consider giving Rh immune globulin. One standard dose protects against the red cells in 30 bags if a maximum red cell contamination value of 0.5 ml/bag is used.[4]

Standard pretransfusion compatibility testing is not done for platelet transfusions. Only documentation of the patient's ABO and Rh is needed to make appropriate selection decisions. Crossmatching is required for single donor platelets containing more than 5 ml red blood cells.[4] HLA typing may be indicated when patients become refractory to platelets after multiple transfusions. The most likely source of compatible donors is the patient's family, although some centers have HLA pre-typed donor files. HLA matching does not guarantee good recovery in alloimmunized patients: no response is seen in 25% of HLA-compatible transfusions.[33] Although many platelet crossmatch procedures are being evaluated for their usefulness as compatibility tests (aggregometry, lymphocytotoxicity, enzyme-linked immunoassay, radioimmunoassay, immunofluorescence and solid-phase testing),[30,33] they are currently used only in research.

Administration

Platelet products must be given through a blood filter. Standard blood infusion sets with 170–220 micron in-line filters may be used. Significant numbers of platelets are not lost in the filter, but a substantial loss can occur from the product volume left in the infusion line.[47] To reduce this loss, special component sets are manufactured with shorter tubing, and small filter surfaces and drip chambers. Very small sets to be used with syringe push infusion are also available. The manufacturer's directions for use must be carefully followed. At one time, it was thought that microaggregate filters were contraindicated for platelet transfusions. Workers have since confirmed that "room temperature" prepared platelets can pass through both screen and depth-type microaggregate filters with little loss, provided they are not occluded with debris and they are rinsed thoroughly with normal saline to clear their priming volume.[7]

To make certain as much product as possible is given, all platelet infusion sets should be flushed with saline after the platelet bag empties by running 20–50 ml through the infusion line. This is easily accomplished with Y-type component infusion sets. Saline rinsing is not indicated for patients with saline or volume restrictions. Transfusion through 18–25 gauge needles does not harm platelets.[48] Platelets may be infused as rapidly as the patient tolerates; infusion rates of 1–2 ml/min[2] up to 5 minutes/bag[49] have been suggested. Platelets may be transfused to infants at rates of 1 ml/min using syringe-type infusion devices.[50]

Reactions

Reactions associated with red cell transfusions are also seen with platelets.[1] Acute hemolytic reactions are very rare complications from ABO-incompatible plasma; infants with small blood volumes are at greatest risk. More commonly seen is the development of a positive direct antiglobulin test, which has little significance to patient well-being. Febrile nonhemolytic and allergic reactions are also common. Fever should not be treated with aspirin, which interferes with platelet function. Of great concern is alloimmunization: 60–70% of patients multiply transfused become sensitized to HLA antigens.[51] Therefore, platelets should only be given for a defined need and in appropriate minimum numbers. Each individual unit carries a disease transmission risk (ie, hepatitis, CMV, AIDS) equal to whole blood. The leukocytes present in platelet products may contribute to the product's sterility during room temperature storage, but rare cases of bacterial contamination have been reported.[33] Both collection and special handling/pooling aspects should be evaluated in these circumstances. The leukocytes may also contribute to graft-versus-host disease (GVHD) in immunocompromised patients.

Granulocytes

Granulocytes are used as supportive therapy in neutropenic patients with sepsis, but their value is uncertain. Transfused granulocytes function normally in vivo and migrate to sites of infection. However, while some groups find improved patient recovery with transfusions, others find no advantage over antibiotic therapy alone. These studies have been reviewed at length.[52–54] Because of the cost and time involved in collecting granulocytes, the adverse reactions experienced by both donors and recipients and the questionable efficacy, the goals of granulocyte transfusion and the criteria for patient selection must be carefully defined.[54]

Most granulocyte transfusions are given to severely neutropenic patients (absolute granulocyte count less than 500/μl) with documented infections that have proven resistant to 1 or 2 days of appropriate, aggressive antibiotic therapy.[14] Candidates should have a reasonable chance of recovery. The effect of transfusion is only temporary and the clinical course of the patient will not change unless the marrow recovers. In a healthy adult, normal daily production of granulocytes in the marrow is 10^{11}, but many times this number are produced in response to infection.[55] Maximum achievable doses in granulocyte transfusion are marginal: 10^{10} given daily for 4 to 6 days or until the patient recovers or the count returns to 500/μl. One hour posttransfusion increments up to 200–500/μl have been reported,[56] but labeling the granulocytes with ^{111}Indium and looking for their sequestration at sites of infection, or simply evaluating patient improvement, are more reliable means of assessing the effect of transfusion.[4]

Although existing neutropenia is an important criterion for selecting candidates for granulocyte transfusion, it need not be a criterion for septic neonates. They are special candidates for granulocyte transfusions for a number of reasons.[57,58] Their stem cell reserve is small and, although stem cells are dividing at a maximum rate, their granulocyte storage pool is small. Cells also take longer to be released from the bone marrow and do not migrate as efficiently. Granulocyte doses of $0.5–1 \times 10^{10}$/kg body weight have been used successfully to treat septic neonates.[59]

A less common use of granulocyte transfusions is in controlling virulent infections in patients with qualitative neutrophil defects, as seen in chronic granulomatous disease and severe burns.[54] Prophylactic use of granulocytes in any patient population is not recommended.

Granulocytes are collected by single donor cytapheresis. Final products should contain approximately 1×10^{10} granulocytes in 200–400 ml plasma. To achieve this number, donors may be pretreated with corticosteroids, and hydroxyethyl starch (HES) is used during the procedure (6–12% of the final product volume may be HES).[1] A considerable number of other leukocytes ($0.1–0.7 \times 10^{10}$), platelets ($20–100 \times 10^{10}$) and red cells (20–50 ml) may also be present in the final product depending on the method of collection.[60] Nylon filtration collection does harvest greater numbers of granulocytes, but it is no longer preferred because of its incidence of associated donor and recipient reactions and reports of impaired granulocyte function.[54]

To supply the smaller doses of granulocytes used in urgent neonatal situations, alternative collection procedures have been developed. Rock et al[61] have separated granulocytes from whole blood less than 24 hours old using HES and centrifugation. The final product contains 1.6×10^9 white cells (75% granulocytes) in 17 ml total volume with a hematocrit of 4%. HES concentration averages 12.6 mg/ml. Goldfinger et al[62] have harvested 1.6×10^9 granulocytes from the fresh red cells remaining after standard plasma and platelet component production using the IBM (Cobe) 2991 Blood Cell Processor.

Storage and Handling

Granulocytes must be transfused as soon as possible after collection, but may be stored up to 24 hours at 20–24 C with no agitation.[4] Chemotactic response is reported to be 87% normal under these conditions. Migration for granulocytes stored at 20–24 C for 8 hours parallels that of fresh granulocytes,[63] but by 24 hours, ability to migrate is significantly reduced. Agitation decreases chemotaxis and bacterial killing functions and increases the hemolysis of red cells present.[64] Granulocytes have been stored frozen up to 18 weeks with 70% survival in experimental studies using a DMSO/HES/albumin cryoprotective solution.[65] Once collected and prepared, granulocyte products are ready for transfusion. If needed for pediatric patients, they may be volume-reduced.

ABO and Rh Compatibility

ABO and Rh antigens are thought not to be present on granulocytes, but because most preparations are heavily contaminated with red cells, ABO-Rh compatibility guidelines parallel those of red cell components (see Appendix 3-1). ABO-identical products are preferred because of the plasma volume. If this is not possible, the red cells in the bag should be ABO-compatible with the recipient's plasma. If the product contains more than 5 ml red cells, it must be ABO-compatible and crossmatched using standard techniques.[3] Rh immune globulin therapy may be indicated when Rh-positive products are given to Rh-negative females who may bear children; one standard dose protects against 15 ml red cells. Current technology does not provide an effective in vitro compatibility test for granulocytes; although many methods exist, no single one detects all relevant antibodies.[66]

Administration

Standard blood infusion sets with 170-micron filters are commonly used for granulocyte transfusion, but component recipient sets may be preferred because of their smaller priming volume. Snyder et al[67] have shown that granulocytes will also pass through screen-type microaggregate filters with only 1–3% retention. Depth-type microaggregate filters retain 20–62% and are therefore contra-indicated. Rinsing the set with normal saline after transfusion flushes out the priming volume but does not appreciably elute the retained granulocytes from the filter. Standard blood needle sizes are appropriate; transfusions have been given through needles as small as 23-gauge, using electromechanical syringe pumps, with no apparent damage.[68]

Granulocytes are transfused slowly over 2 to 4 hours to minimize transfusion reactions, and patients should be closely monitored. Pretreatment with antihistamines, nonaspirin antipyretics, meperidine injections and steroids may be necessary to manage reactions.[4] Neonates appear to tolerate granulocyte transfusion much better than adults; the literature is surprisingly free of adverse reactions in this patient group even at infusion rates of 10^9 granulocytes/15 ml/kg body weight in 30–45 minutes.[57]

Reactions

Hemolytic transfusion reactions are possible with granulocyte transfusions, but they can be avoided by using ABO-compatible components. Allergic reactions have also been reported. Febrile nonhemolytic reactions caused by leukocyte antibody-antigen interactions are seen in 5–15% of patients transfused depending on the method of product preparation.[56] Patients with lung infections are at special risk of developing severe pulmonary reactions with shortness of breath, cough and usually fever. The etiology of these reactions is not clear, but contributing factors include fluid overload, localization of infused granulocytes at the site of infection and toxic reactions causing granulocyte degranulation, adherence of cells to endothelium and complement activation.[52] Leukoagglutinins causing aggregation and embolization of granulocytes in the lungs present a similar picture and may be the most severe of all. Amphotericin B, given for fungal infections, increases granulocyte aggregation and exacerbates pulmonary reactions.[54]

Like red cell components and platelets, granulocytes can alloimmunize patients, transmit diseases like hepatitis, CMV and AIDS, and cause GVHD. This is especially important to bone marrow transplant recipients who are at risk for CMV and GVHD and who, in their course of treatment, might be considered candidates for granulocyte transfusions.

Plasma Products

The use of plasma (fresh frozen and single donor) has increased tenfold in the United States over the past 10 years to reach a total of 2 million units transfused annually. To evaluate this increase, a

National Institutes of Health (NIH) Consensus Conference was convened in September, 1984. Panel members concluded that few definitive indications for plasma exist, that many patients can be managed more effectively and safely with alternative treatment, and made specific recommendations[69]:

1. Plasma should *not* be used as a volume expander; crystalloid solutions, colloid solutions with albumin, HES, or Dextran can be given with less risk and expense.
2. Plasma should *not* be used as a source of nutrition; hyperalimentation (amino-acid) solutions and dextrose are preferred.
3. Plasma *is* indicated to replace coagulation factor deficiencies that have no specific factor concentrate available, or where concentrate use in a given situation is less effective or safe. Plasma *may* be indicated in other situations not fully supported by data.

Indications

Proposed indications have been discussed at length[69-71] and will only be briefly summarized below.

Coagulation Factor Replacement

Bleeding related to congenital or acquired deficiencies in coagulation Factors II, V, VII, IX, X and XI can be treated with plasma transfusions. Concentrates are available for Factors II, VII, IX and X; but, because they carry a high risk of hepatitis and thrombosis, plasma is preferred unless the total volume needed is too great. Plasma is the only product available for Factors V and XI replacement; congenital deficiencies in these two factors are very rare.

The most common users of plasma for replacement of Factors II, VII, IX and X are patients with liver disease.[71] Their disease may reduce factor synthesis, induce episodes of consumptive coagulapathy and increase risk of bleeding from complications of esophageal varices and portal hypertension. Plasma transfusion is definitely needed if the patient is bleeding. Need is less clear if the patient is not bleeding, but will be surgically challenged. Prothrombin time (PT) and partial thromboplastin time (PTT) results are poor predictors of surgical bleeding, and abnormal test results are difficult to correct. Stable patients not being challenged do not need transfusion. Concentrate use is contraindicated in liver disease because of the high risk of DIC and thrombosis.[72]

Coumarin Drug Reversal

Coumarin drugs stop the production of functional Factors II, VII, IX and X. If a patient on coumarin drugs starts to bleed or is scheduled for surgery, the effect of the drug can be reversed with vitamin K injections: a dose of 10–30 mg will correct factor deficiency in 6–12 hours.[71] These factors all have different rates of synthesis, which affect the rate of their return to hemostatic levels. Therefore, both the PT and PTT, tests that adequately assess all factors, are recommended for following coumarin reversal.[73] If time is urgent, plasma is the treatment of choice.

Massive Transfusion

Dilution of coagulation factors in massive transfusion settings (greater than one blood volume in 24 hours) is very uncommon,[9] even when red cells are transfused instead of whole blood. Factor levels may decrease, but they rarely drop below 25–30%. Most factors equilibrate into the extravascular space, which serves as a reserve pool and compensates for any potential dilution. Even Factor VIII rarely drops below 50%: Factor VIII bound to the vascular endothelium is released under stress to provide an additional reserve. Unless there is a coexisting DIC or other medical condition, factor support is not needed. Platelets, which are largely intravascular, become diluted with massive transfusion and may be needed.[9] The coagulation factors present in platelet plasma are considerable and help contribute to hemostasis.[36]

Abnormal PT and PTT results are difficult to correct in massive transfusion. If plasma is needed in hemorrhagic shock, large volumes (600–2000 ml) must be given quickly (over 1 to 2 hours) to effect any significant improvement.[70]

Antithrombin III Deficiency

Antithrombin III (AT III) is a major inhibitor of coagulation factors, especially thrombin.[74] Patients deficient in AT III are at risk of thrombosis, and heparin, often used in the treatment of thrombosis, will not work without AT III. AT III concentrates are available in Europe, but are only used experimentally in the United States and carry an increased risk of hepatitis.[75] Plasma is given in place of concentrates to patients with congenital deficiencies or acquired deficiencies (from liver disease, oral contraceptives, nephrosis, DIC, diabetes, sepsis, eclampsia and some drugs) when they are scheduled for surgery or require heparin treatment.[75]

Immunodeficiencies

Plasma can be a source of immunoglobulins for primary humoral deficiencies, and for secondary deficiencies in infants with severe protein-losing enteropathies who do not respond to total parenteral nutrition. However, purified immune globulin for intravenous use is preferred.[69,71]

Thrombotic Thrombocytopenic Purpura

Thrombotic thrombocytopenic purpura (TTP) is a poorly understood disorder that is characterized by platelet aggregates in terminal arterioles. Multiple etiologies may be responsible, including an increase of some platelet aggregation factor or a deficiency in some platelet aggregation inhibitor.[76] Therapeutic plasma exchange with fresh frozen plasma, used in conjunction with antiplatelet agents, corticosteroids and plasma infusions, has proven effective in controlling thrombotic episodes.[77] The benefits of using fresh frozen plasma over single donor plasma are not known.[71]

Fresh Frozen Plasma

Plasma separated from whole blood and placed in frozen storage at -18 C within 6 hours of collection is known as fresh frozen plasma (FFP). The total volume averages 200–250 ml and includes a portion of the anticoagulant. FFP contains optimal levels of *all* plasma clotting factors: 0.7–1 unit factor activity per ml or approximately 200 units factor activity per bag, and 200–400 mg fibrinogen per bag.[1] FFP is the most common plasma product available to transfusion services and is appropriate for all the indications discussed above.

Hemostatic doses may be calculated using the patient's blood volume plus current and desired factor levels, or may be estimated: 10 ml/kg body weight provides a hemostatic dose for most factors for both adults and infants.[2(p 19)] The frequency of transfusion depends on what factors are being replaced, their half-life, and the patient's clinical course. Initial doses are generally higher (>15 ml/kg) than maintenance doses. Factors are compared in Table 3-3. FFP should be transfused only with a defined need. Following laboratory PT and PTT results may be helpful in some situations. If normal results are found in a patient with active bleeding, problems other than factor deficiencies should be considered. However, abnormal test results by themselves do not predict the patient will bleed.

Table 3-3. Coagulation Factors[4,78]

Factor	% Needed for Hemostasis	In Vivo Half-Life	Stability in Blood Stored at 4 C
I	(70–100 mg/dl)	3–5 days	Stable
II	?20–40	3 days	Stable
V	15–25	?12–36 hours	Labile
VII	5–10	4–6 hours	Stable
VIII	25–30	11–14 hours	Labile
IX	?15–25	24–32 hours	Stable
X	10–20	24–60 hours	Stable
XI	?10	48–84 hours	?Stable
XIII	2–3	6–10 days[79]	Stable

Single Donor Plasma

Single donor plasma (SDP) is a generic term for plasma that does not meet the rigid standards of fresh frozen. It comes from a number of sources: plasma separated from whole blood before 5 days after the whole blood expires, fresh frozen plasma in frozen storage that was not used within its 1-year expiration time or fresh frozen plasma that was thawed and not used within 24 hours of thawing.[4] The final volume and content of SDP is similar to FFP, except that it may be deficient in Factor V and VIII levels and, if prepared from stored whole blood, may have higher levels of potassium and ammonia.[4] If prepared from modified whole blood, cryoprecipitate removed, it will be deficient in fibrinogen as well, but will be labeled as such. SDP may be used in place of FFP for all indications discussed above except Factor V replacement and TTP. In some geographical regions, SDP is used more as a source for albumin and immune serum globulin production, and therefore is not always available to the transfusion service.

Storage and Handling

FFP is stored frozen at temperatures colder than −18 C up to 1 year from the date of collection. Before it can be transfused, it is thawed in a 30–37 C waterbath with gentle agitation or kneading; to provide maximum benefit to the patient, all precipitates must be resuspended. This thawing process takes approximately 30 minutes. Waterbaths may be contaminated with bacteria. To avoid contaminating the area around the bag's sterile entry ports, a plastic overwrap may be used.[80] After thawing, FFP is stored at 1–6 C until it is issued for transfusion. It must be transfused within 24 hours after thawing according to AABB *Standards*[3] and within 6 hours according to the FDA. Because of these time limits, FFP is thawed preferably just before use, and the new expiration is indicated on the label. If the product cannot be issued within this time, the FFP is relabeled SDP and can still be given to patients who do not need labile coagulation Factors V and VIII.

ABO and Rh Compatibility

Compatibility testing is not done for plasma transfusions. However, the patient's ABO group must be known prior to product selection to make sure A or B antibodies in the plasma are compatible with the patient's red cells (see Appendix 3-1). This is especially important to infants with small blood volumes. If the patient's group is not known, group AB FFP can be safely given. Plasma bags may be labeled with the donor's Rh type, but Rh is not considered in their selection.

Administration

Standard blood infusion sets or special component infusion sets with in-line 170 micron filters are used for plasma transfusions. As with platelet transfusions, it is good practice to rinse the bag and infusion line with normal saline after the transfusion so the priming volume is not wasted. Y-type infusion sets simplify this rinse process. Microaggregate filter sets may also be used, but they offer no advantages and have a larger priming volume to flush. Manufacturers' directions should always be carefully followed and the patient's chart must be checked for saline and volume restrictions. Needles appropriate for red cell transfusions may be used for plasma products, but smaller sizes may be preferred if the patient has a known bleeding problem. Infusion should proceed as fast as the patient tolerates; rates of 4–10 ml/min have been suggested.[1,49] Most transfusions are completed within 1 to 2 hours.

Reactions

Chills, fever and allergic reactions may occur with plasma transfusions. Severe allergic reactions with pulmonary complications are possible if the donor has antibodies to the patient's leukocytes. Circulatory overload may occur with fast infusion rates. Hemolytic reactions are rare and generally mild; a positive direct antiglobulin test may develop if antibodies in the plasma react with the recipient's red cells. Plasma, like all other blood components, has a risk of disease transmission similar to whole blood. If very large volumes of plasma are transfused, hypothermia and citrate toxicity are possible, especially in infants.[81]

Cryoprecipitate

When FFP is thawed at 4 C, a white cold-insoluble precipitate forms. This material, which is separated from the plasma and refrozen, is the product cryoprecipitate. One bag contains 80–120 units of VIII:C (Factor VIII procoagulant activity), 40–70% of von Willebrand's Factor (vWF) and 20–30% of the Factor XIII present in the initial plasma, 150–250 mg fibrinogen, and about 55 mg fibronectin,[82] all suspended in 10–15 ml plasma.[2,4] The primary use of cryoprecipitate is to control bleeding associated with a deficiency or defect in one of the coagulation factors listed above; however, additional applications have been reported. Appropriate uses are summarized below.

Hemophilia A

Hemophilia A is a congenital hereditary bleeding disorder caused by a deficiency in coagulation Factor VIII:C. Normal Factor VIII:C activity ranges from 50–150%. This percent activity refers to the amount of coagulation factor in the sample compared to fresh, normal pooled plasma, which has 1 unit/ml or 100% activity. Individuals with severe hemophilia A have less than 1% activity and may bleed spontaneously. Those with mild hemophilia A have greater than 5% activity and may only bleed with trauma or surgery. Bleeding can be managed with cryoprecipitate transfusions; doses are calculated using laboratory data[4]:

\# Cryo bags needed = total Factor VIII units needed/80 units Factor VIII per bag

where total Factor VIII units needed =

Plasma volume × (% desired activity − % initial activity)

and plasma volume =

(kg body weight × 70 ml/kg) − (1 − hematocrit)

High purity Factor VIII concentrates may be used in place of cryoprecipitate; however, they carry an increased risk of hepatitis. Cryoprecipitate may be preferred, especially for the very young, as long as it can supply sufficient Factor VIII. Because the amount of Factor VIII:C in cryoprecipitate is variable, a minimum of 3 bags is pooled for small doses.[75]

Minimum Factor VIII levels of 20% are recommended for treatment of early hemorrhage, 30–50% for established hemorrhage.[83] Activity levels greater than 50% are preferred for major surgery. Initial doses should be large enough to raise the activity level to twice the minimum level. The initial half-life of infused Factor VIII:C is 4 hours because of equilibration.[83] Thereafter, the biologic half-life is 8–12 hours. When levels drop to the minimum (every 12 hours), half doses are given to maintain activity above the minimum. Dose and length of treatment vary with the extent of surgery and the bleed, the rate of healing and Factor VIII:C assays. Treatment may continue for several weeks.

Von Willebrand's Disease

Von Willebrand's disease (vWD) is another hereditary bleeding disorder related to a deficiency or abnormality in von Willebrand's Factor (vWF), a high-molecular weight, multimeric glycoprotein that promotes platelet adherence to subendothelium collagen and the formation of the platelet plug. VWF associates with Factor VIII in circulation and may help to stabilize it; patients with vWD may have concurrent deficiencies in Factor VIII:C. Several genetic variants in the disease have been identified[83]: Type I, a quantitative deficiency of normal multimers that may be due to a defect in their mechanism of release into circulation; Type II, a defect in synthesis and assembly of vWF such that large multimers are missing; and Type III, a severe, possibly recessive condition clinically similar to severe hemophilia A.

Cryoprecipitate is the blood component of choice for treating bleeding episodes in vWD. Patients require both vWF and Factor VIII:C activity for hemostasis, and cryoprecipitate is a concentrate of both in a small usable volume. Factor VIII concentrates lose much of their vWF during processing and are not recommended. Cryoprecipitate dose depends on clinical and laboratory severity of the disease and the nature and severity of the bleed: single doses of 1 bag/6–10 kg body weight have been used.[75,83] Patient response is monitored clinically and with bleeding times. After cryoprecipitate infusions, vWF levels immediately rise as expected, then begin to decline with a half-life of 8–12 hours. The bleeding time may return to baseline a few hours postinfusion, perhaps because of preferential clearance of the larger, more effective vWF multimers.[84] Patients with vWD Type I have also been successfully treated with the drug desmopressin acetate (DDVAP), which mediates the release of vWF and Factor VIII:C from vascular endothelial cells.[83] This drug may also benefit patients with mild hemophilia A.

Factor XIII Deficiency

Individuals with severe hereditary Factor XIII deficiency present with bleeding from the umbilical cord during the first few days of life and may suffer lifelong from episodes of ecchymoses, hematomas, prolonged bleeding following trauma and poor wound healing.[85] The long biological half-life of Factor XIII, coupled with the very low levels required for hemostasis (2–3%), make bleeding episodes easy to treat. Factor XIII is stable in all plasma products, but it is concentrated 4–6 times in cryoprecipitate. Doses of one bag cryoprecipitate per 10–20 kg body weight infused every 3–4 weeks have been recommended.[2,4] Factor XIII is also decreased in DIC and liver disease, but not sufficiently so to cause symptoms.

Fibrinogen Deficiency

Normal fibrinogen levels are 200–400 mg/dl; only 70–100 mg/dl are needed for hemostasis.[78] Decreased levels in DIC, liver disease and congenital afibrinogenemia or hypofibrinogenemia, when associated with bleeding, are preferentially treated with cryoprecipitate. Fibrinogen assays are helpful in calculating the appropriate dose using formulas similar to those for Factor VIII:

Total fibrinogen needed =
Plasma volume × (Desired fibrinogen level −
Initial fibrinogen level)

To simplify ordering in emergency situations, a single transfusion dose of eight bags of cryoprecipitate (2 g fibrinogen) has been suggested.[2 (p 23)] Patients with congenital and acquired dysfibrinogenemia facing surgical challenge or acutely bleeding may also require cryoprecipitate transfusion.

Fibronectin Deficiency

Fibronectin is a glycoprotein that acts as a cellular glue: it is involved in cell-to-cell adhesion, and helps remove foreign matter and bacteria from blood by mediating their attachment to phagocytic cells. Normal plasma values are 180–720 μg/ml (males) and 150–540 μg/ml (females).[86] Following major surgery, trauma or burns, these levels decrease.[87] Saba et al[88,89] used cryoprecipitate to treat fibronectin deficiencies in septic injured patients and reported marked clinical improvement in bacteriological, hematological and pulmonary functions.

Although its small volume makes cryoprecipitate the component of choice for treatment, recent investigations have confirmed that fibronectin is stable in whole blood, single donor plasma, fresh frozen plasma and platelets, as well as cryoprecipitate, with little degradation.[82] Because very ill patients are frequently transfused with many of these products, total transfusion requirements should be considered when assessing the need and component of choice for fibronectin replacement.

Uremic Bleeding

A variety of hemostatic disorders and abnormal bleeding tendencies are associated with uremia. Dialysis has been used to reduce the frequency of bleeding; platelet transfusions produce only temporary improvement. Neither therapy is uniformly effective. Cryoprecipitate transfusions (10 bags/dose) have been tried with apparent success.[90] Bleeding times shortened within one to several hours and remained shortened for 24 hours. Abnormal bleeding times associated with storage pool disease have also been corrected with cryoprecipitate.[91] The mechanism of action in both of these situations is unclear.

Removal of Renal Calculi

Surgically removing small renal calculi can be a troublesome challenge: small free-floating stones, fragments and amorphous material can be left behind to serve as a nucleus for more stone growth and recurrent problems.[92] Simultaneous injection of cryoprecipitate, thrombin and calcium chloride into the renal pelvis produces an extremely strong gel that can be pulled out with forceps, carrying trapped particles with it. Three or four bags of cryoprecipitate may be needed for the procedure, depending on the volume capacity of the renal pelvis and calyceal system.[92,93]

Storage and Handling

After preparation from fresh frozen plasma, cryoprecipitate is stored frozen at temperatures colder than -18 C up to 1 year from the date of the initial whole blood donation. Immediately before use, it is thawed in a 30–37 C waterbath. Using a plastic overwrap or drying the entry ports with a clean, dry towel or gauze is again recommended to prevent the bath water from contaminating the contents with bacteria when the bag is entered for pooling or transfusion.[80] Thawing occurs rapidly (about 10 minutes) because of the small volume of the product. After thawing, cryoprecipitate is stored at room temperature up to 6 hours. The new expiration time is written on the label.

To simplify administration, transfusion services will pool the contents of all the bags ordered into a transfer bag or syringe. This pooling process takes another 15 minutes. Before pooling, the products should be mixed well with their suspending media. Sterile normal saline may be used to help rinse the bags completely of their content. Once pooled, FDA recommends that the product expire in 4 hours.

Pools of 2–6 cryoprecipitate bags can be prepared in advance and stored frozen up to 1 year, providing aseptic technique is used and the label reflects the 4-hour expiration after thawing.[4] These "Cryoprecipitate, Pooled" products will also be labeled with the plasma or saline volume used in pooling.

ABO and Rh Compatibility

Cryoprecipitate is essentially free of red cells, but it commonly has a very small volume of plasma and, therefore, ABO antibodies. The plasma of products selected for transfusion should be ABO-compatible with the patient's red cells, especially for patients with small blood volumes (see Appendix 3-1).[3] Compatibility testing is not done, but the patient's ABO group must be known in advance to make the appropriate selection. If the patient's group is not known, group AB is preferred. In emergencies, any group may be given because the plasma volume is very small. Rh matching is not needed.

Some suppliers prepare "dry" cryoprecipitate with almost all plasma removed. These products are labeled with their ABO group, but can be given without considering ABO compatibility. Infusionists should consult their transfusion service or blood supplier for local recommendations.

Administration

Cellular material from leukocytes, platelets and red cells, plus fibrin and amorphous protein have been reported in cryoprecipitate; therefore, the product must be transfused through a filter.[94] Standard blood and special component infusion sets with in-line 170 micron filters are most commonly used. It is common practice to flush the infusion set with 20–30 ml sterile normal saline following transfusion to prevent the loss of the priming volume, provided the patient is not volume- or saline-restricted. Sets with small priming volumes are preferred. Needle guidelines for red cell components and plasma products are appropriate for cryoprecipitate.

Cryoprecipitates should be transfused as rapidly as the patient can tolerate: rates of 4–10 ml/min have been suggested.[1,49] One group recommends that if a syringe method of administration is used, undue pressure on the syringe be avoided, because this may increase the amount of particulate matter transfused and contribute to allergic reactions.[94]

Reactions

When ABO-incompatible cryoprecipitate is given, a weakly positive DAT may develop, and with very high doses, hemolysis may be seen. Febrile and allergic reactions are also possible. The incidence of disease transmission (eg, hepatitis, AIDS) for each unit transfused is similar to that of whole blood.

Plasma Derivatives

Large pools of donor plasma can be fractionated into more purified protein products called plasma derivatives using the cold ethanol precipitation principle developed by Edwin Cohn. His basic procedure used the variables of ethanol concentration, protein concentration, ionic strength, pH and temperature to separate albumin and the gammaglobulins.[95] If the starting product is FFP, a cryoprecipitate may be separated first, then purified and concentrated into Factor VIII concentrates by a number of different methods. Concentrates of Factors II, VII, IX and X (known as Prothrombin Complex Concentrates) can also be made from plasma before fractionation, using their affinity to adsorb to certain chemicals or ion exchangers.

These derivatives contain no cellular elements and are given without regard to ABO or Rh compatibility. No serological testing need be documented on the patient before infusion. Therefore, they are more frequently dispensed by the pharmacy department than by the transfusion service.

Albumin/Plasma Protein Fractions

Although only 60% of the plasma protein content is albumin, it supplies 80% of plasma's oncotic activity and is the principal product of fractionation. It is commercially available as plasma protein fraction (PPF), which has a protein content of 83% albumin/17% alpha and beta globulin and as more purified 5% and 25% albumin, which have protein contents of 96% albumin/4% globulin. All three products have sodium levels of approximately 145 mEq/l.[2] They may contain stabilizers to preserve albumin polymers during the fractionation process, but they have no preservatives.

Patients receiving albumin should be both hypovolemic and hypoproteinemic because these products provide fast volume expansion and colloid replacement. PPF and 5% albumin are osmotically equivalent to an equal volume of plasma and are used interchangeably. 25% albumin, being 5 times more concentrated, is osmotically equivalent to 5 times its volume of plasma. Because it will pull water out of the extravascular space so effectively, 25% albumin must not be given to dehydrated patients without supplemental fluids, or to patients at risk of circulatory overload.[2]

Albumin is used to correct large, acute losses of colloid as seen in hypovolemic shock from trauma or surgery; up to 500 ml may be given and the patient's response evaluated. For severe burns, doses are calculated to keep the plasma protein level above 5.2 g/dl. Albumin therapy will not affect the long-term albumin deficiencies associated with chronic liver disease, chronic nephrosis and other protein-losing enteropathies, but it may be indicated in individual cases to support blood pressure during hypotensive episodes, or induce diuresis in fluid overload. Appropriate uses are more thoroughly reviewed elsewhere.[96-98] Albumin products should not be used to correct nutritional hypoproteinemia because they lack some essential amino acids and take several weeks to degrade.[96]

Storage and Handling

Albumin products stored at room temperature (not greater than 37 C) may be used up to 3 years from the date of manufacturing. If stored at 2–8 C, they may be used up to 5 years. These products are supplied in glass bottles, which may develop cracks if frozen and permit the entry of bacteria. Therefore, manufacturers recommend the solution be inspected before infusion and discarded if it appears to have been frozen or appears turbid. Manufacturers also recommend the product be used within 4 hours of opening, and that unused portions be discarded to reduce the risk of contamination. Albumin is ready to use with no further preparation.

Administration

Blood transfusion sets/filters are not needed for infusing albumin and PPF; equipment appropriate for any USP infusion solution is used instead. Some manufacturers supply the infusion set, with or without attached needle, with drip chamber and air check valve. They recommend the top be swabbed with an antiseptic before the bottle is spiked. Albumin products must never be allowed to mix with amino acid or protein solutions in the line because this may cause the proteins to precipitate.[98] 25% albumin should also not be mixed with red cells because it is hypertonic. Although 5% albumin is used with red cell transfusions, PPF has been reported to produce unacceptable hemolysis when mixed with older packed cells.[99]

When given to patients with reduced blood volumes, 5% and 25% albumin may be given as rapidly as the patient tolerates. When the blood volume is normal or only slightly reduced, rates of 2–4 ml/min have been suggested for 5%, and 1 ml/min for 25%.[98] Children are infused at ½ to ¼ this adult rate. More caution is used when infusing PPF. Hypotension may occur with rates greater than 10 ml/min; therefore, blood pressure should be monitored carefully during the infusion, and the infusion slowed or stopped according to patient response. PPF should not be given intraarterially.

Reactions

Adverse reactions to albumin products are rare, but allergic symptoms (flushing, urticaria, fever, chills and headache) have all been reported. If albumin is given too quickly, circulatory overload problems and pulmonary edema may develop. 25% albumin may also complicate interstitial dehydration. Giving daily doses of 150 g/day may decrease globulin, fibrinogen and coagulation factor synthesis.[4]

Severe hypotensive episodes have been reported with rapid infusions of PPF.[96,97] The vasodilation has been implicated with PPF's acetate buffer and with prekallikrein activators, precursors to bradykinin. Bradykinin is a potent hypotensive agent that is inactivated in the lungs; therefore, PPF should not be used when rapid infusion is needed, or when the lungs are bypassed, ie, intraarterial infusions or cardiopulmonary bypass procedures. Similar hypotensive reactions have been reported with albumin, but this is much more rare.

Albumin products have not been reported to transmit hepatitis or AIDS. They are heat-treated at 60 C for 10 hours to reduce the risk of hepatitis transmission. Recent data suggest that the steps involved in large-scale plasma fractionation (cold ethanol, low pH) also reduce the risk of HTLV-III transmission.[100]

Immune Serum Globulin

Immune serum globulin (ISG) is a concentrated solution of gamma globulin made from large pools of normal human plasma. When donors with high-titered antibodies to a specific disease are used in the pool, a hyperimmune product is produced. The standard ISG solution from fractionation contains approximately 16 g/dl protein: 95–98% is IgG, and 1–2% IgM and IgA.[2,98] Because IgG aggregates that form during the manufacturing process are capable of activating complement and producing anaphylactic shock if given intra-venously, standard ISG solutions must be given intramuscularly. Recently, several technologies (reduction-alkylation, pepsin diges-tion and polyethylene glycol precipitation) have been used to remove IgG aggregates from ISG.[101] Although these new ISG preparations are quite expensive and contain only 5 g/dl protein, they can be given intravenously, which offers some clinical advantages. They are preferred for patients with small muscle mass, those who expe-rience severe pain from injections and patients with bleeding ten-dencies. Intravenous gamma globulin (IV-IgG) also makes "high-dose therapy" possible.[101]

ISG is used to provide prophylactic passive antibody to suscep-tible individuals who have been exposed to a specific disease (eg, rubella, tetanus, hepatitis, varicella-zoster). If a hyperimmune prod-uct is available, it is the product of choice. To be most effective, it should be given as quickly after exposure as possible, before the virus infects the host cells. The dose depends on the disease, the globulin product and body weight. The manufacturer's directions should be consulted. ISG is also used as replacement therapy in congenital immunoglobulin deficiencies. To maintain immunoglob-ulin levels of greater than 200 mg%, monthly doses of 0.7 ml stan-dard ISG/kg body weight or 100 mg (2ml) IV-Ig G/kg are given.[2]

Rh Immune Globulin (RHIG), purified anti-D, is a special ISG product. It is given to Rh-negative individuals who have been exposed to Rh-positive red cells through pregnancy or transfusion to prevent their becoming sensitized to the D antigen. Two RHIG doses are currently available in the United States: a standard or full dose, which protects the recipient from 30 ml whole blood, and a "mini" dose, which protects from exposure to 5 ml whole blood. These products are licensed for intramuscular injection only, although intravenous products are available outside the United States. Indi-cations of use and proper determination of dose are summarized elsewhere.[4]

High-dose, IV-IgG therapy has been successfully used in the management of idiopathic thrombocytopenic purpura (ITP). ITP is an autoimmune disease characterized by increased destruction of platelets. This is due to platelet antibody attachment and subse-quent platelet removal by the reticuloendothelial (RE) system. Patients experience petechiae, purpura and, rarely, serious bleed-ing. Cases that do not go into spontaneous remission are treated with splenectomy. High-dose, IV-IgG offers an alternative treat-ment: a dose of 1–2 g/kg given over several days will stop bleeding and restore hemostasis. The IgG presumably blocks platelet removal by the RE system, although its precise role has yet to be defined.

The product IV-IgG, its mechanisms of action and its applications have been recently reviewed.[101]

ISG/IV-IgG should not be used to treat recurrent infections without a known deficiency, or chronic stable ITP conditions. It is contraindicated for patients who have known systemic reactions to ISG infusion or antibodies to IgA.

Storage and Handling

Immune serum globulin products may be stored at 2–8 C up to 3 years from the date of manufacture, depending on the specific product. Freezing may further aggregate IgG molecules; therefore, vials that have been frozen should be discarded. Most products are supplied as a solution ready to use. One commercially available IV-IgG comes freeze-dried and must be resuspended according to manufacturer's directions before use. Products should be used promptly after opening, and unused portions should be discarded.

Administration

Great care must be taken to administer the product by its correct route: standard ISG must be given intramuscularly and IV-IgG must be given intravenously. Manufacturers recommend that IV-IgG be given through a separate infusion line to avoid its mixing with other solutions. Infusion rates should begin slowly, 0.01–0.02 ml/kg for the first 30 minutes. If no problems occur, the rate may be increased to 0.02–0.04 ml/kg/min.[98] The patient should be monitored carefully throughout the infusion and epinephrine should be readily available in case acute anaphylactic symptoms develop.

Reactions

The most common reaction to intramuscular ISG is local tenderness and muscle stiffness at the site of injection. Systemic reactions with urticaria, flushing, headache, fever and angioedema have also been reported. Anaphylactic reactions are rare. Symptoms may result from the stabilizers and preservatives in the product, as well as the protein itself.[96,101]

Manufacturers report that reactions from IV-IgG are mild or moderate with headache being the most common symptom, and emesis, chills, fever, chest tightness and nausea reported less frequently. Many symptoms, including anxiety, flushing, chills, wheezing, back pain, dizziness and general malaise, are rate-dependent. True anaphylactic reactions are rare and often associated with a history of severe allergic reactions to plasma products.

ISG preparations contain low titers of ABO antibodies; other alloantibodies such as anti-D have also been detected. When large amounts are administered, these antibodies may cause a positive DAT and subsequent hemolysis.[102]

There is low or no risk of hepatitis and AIDS transmission from ISG products even though they are not heat-treated as are the albumin products. Depending on the fractionation process, hepatitis B virus tends not to coprecipitate with Cohn Fraction II from which ISG is made. Any residual virus may be eliminated by the concentrated antibodies in the solution. The risk of AIDS infectivity is also thought to be reduced or eliminated from the basic manufacturing process using cold ethanol and low pH.[100] Transmission of non-A,non-B hepatitis has been reported with IV-IgG and may be postulated with ISG, perhaps because the level of antibody in the general population is lower.[103]

Factor VIII Concentrate

Factor VIII:C can be purified from the cold insoluble fraction of pooled FFP, then lyophilized into a concentrated product that is easy to store, transport and transfuse. Because of their availability, ease of use and small volume, concentrates have replaced cryoprecipitate as the product of choice to control bleeding in individuals with severe hemophilia A. Every vial is labeled with its total Factor VIII:C activity, which may vary from 250–1500 units depending on concentration and vial size. Doses are easily calculated by dividing the total number of Factor VIII:C units needed (see formula on page 68) by the total number of units per vial. A simpler dose estimation can be made by assuming that 1 unit Factor VIII:C infused per kg body weight will produce a 2% rise in plasma level.[98] Factor VIII concentrates also contain some fibrinogen and vWF, but not enough to warrant their use for these factor deficiencies.

Factor VIII concentrates available today are heat-treated. This processing was developed in an effort to reduce the high incidence of hepatitis associated with their use. The additional heating does not appear to be effective against hepatitis, but it does appear to be helpful in reducing the risk of HTLV-III infectivity.[75,83] Because of concern over the growing number of hemophiliacs who are seropositive for HTLV-III, the National Hemophilia Foundation's Medical and Scientific Advisory Committee now recommends heat-treated concentrates as the preferred product for all severe hemophiliacs, although they acknowledge cryoprecipitate as an acceptable alternative in regions with a low prevalence of AIDS.[104] Because of its lower risk of hepatitis, cryoprecipitate may be preferred for very young or newly diagnosed hemophiliacs who have not yet been transfused.

Storage and Handling

Lyophilized Factor VIII:C is stored at 2–8 C up to 1 year from the date of manufacture; however, it may also be kept up to 3 months at room temperature. Like the other plasma derivatives stored in glass bottles, Factor VIII:C should not be frozen. Just before use, it must be reconstituted following the manufacturer's directions. The diluent is frequently supplied along with the concentrate. Manufacturers recommend reconstituted Factor VIII be infused within 3 hours of reconstitution to avoid problems from bacterial contamination.

Administration

The common method of infusion is intravenously by direct syringe injection; plastic syringes are preferred over glass. Even though solutions must be completely dissolved before infusion, they will still contain particulate matter; therefore, manufacturers may supply special filter needles in addition to the diluent. One group of investigators has found that this material passes through standard 170-micron filters and concluded that it may be responsible for pulmonary function changes observed after concentrate injections.[105] Forty-micron filters can effectively remove the debris. If large volumes are to be given, drip infusion methods may also be used.

When more than 34 units of Factor VIII:C per ml are being given, maximum infusion rates of 2 ml/min are recommended. When less concentrated solutions are being given, 10–20 ml may be infused over 3 minutes.[98] Vital signs should be monitored during the infusion. If the patient responds with an adverse change in vital signs, eg, an increase in pulse, the infusion rate should be slowed.

Reactions

Allergic reactions may result from infusions of Factor VIII concentrates, with symptoms of bronchospasm, urticaria, fever, chills, nausea, headache, vomiting and general malaise. Acute symptoms of erythema, fever and backache occur infrequently and usually disappear within 20 minutes.[98] Because anti-A and anti-B are present in concentrates, a positive DAT may develop postinfusion and, rarely, acute hemolysis is seen following large-dose infusions when the patient is group A, B or AB. Hyperfibrinogenemia may also be seen after high-dose therapy. The significance of this is questionable, but it may put the patient in a hypercoaguable state. The greatest concern in concentrate use is the risk of hepatitis transmission. One study reported 90% of individuals treated with Factor VIII:C concentrates show serological evidence of a past or present HBV infection.[106]

Factor IX Concentrates

Factor IX Concentrates are also called Prothrombin Complex Concentrates (PCC) because, in addition to Factor IX, they contain other factors within the prothrombin complex: Factors II, X, variable amounts of VII and Protein C.[75] These are separated from pooled plasma and lyophilized and bottled into a product similar to Factor VIII concentrates. One vial contains 500–1000 units of Factor IX and reconstitutes into a 20–40 ml volume, depending on the manufacturer. The factor assay in units/vial is given on the label.

The primary use of PCC is to control bleeding in individuals with severe hemophilia B, a congenital hereditary deficiency of coagulation Factor IX. Normal activity levels of Factor IX are 50–180% (the level in 1 ml fresh normal pooled plasma being 1 unit or 100%); hemostasis is well-maintained with levels above 25%.[83] Patients with severe hemophilia B have levels less than 1% and present with spontaneous bleeding into joints and muscles much like patients with severe hemophilia A. Infusing 1 unit/kg body weight will raise the Factor IX activity level 1%,[83] but, as with Factor VIII, initial loading doses must be larger than maintenance doses because only 30–50% Factor IX is seen in circulation immediately posttransfusion. The rest equilibrates into the extravascular space. The biological half-life is 32 hours; therefore, transfusion may be needed only once or twice a week until hemostasis is controlled.[83]

Some of the factors in PCC are activated during the manufacturing process. This characteristic has made it useful in treating patients with hemophilia A and Factor VIII inhibitors. Approximately 15% of hemophiliacs develop a neutralizing antibody to Factor VIII; some antibodies rise to very high titers with Factor VIII infusions, making hemostasis almost impossible to achieve. The activated factors in PCC help bypass the need for Factor VIII in the coagulation scheme, although their precise mechanism of action is not clear.[75] Infusions of 75 units of Factor IX/kg may be given every 12 hours for two to three doses in an attempt to control bleeding in these "high responding inhibitor" situations.[75]

Activated PCC, a product with higher levels of activated factors, is now being manufactured specifically for patients with high responding inhibitors to Factor VIII or Factor IX. These products are very expensive and their increased effectiveness is controversial.[75]

Multi-factor deficiencies of Factors II, VII, IX and X seen in liver disease, vitamin K deficiency, malabsorption syndromes and coumarin therapy and congenital factor deficiencies are not treated with PCC because of its increased risk of disease transmission (eg, hepatitis) and its high association with thrombosis. FFP transfusions are preferred.[4] PCC should not be used if there is evidence of DIC.

Storage and Handling

Factor IX concentrates may be stored up to 1 year from the date of manufacturing at 2–8 C, but room temperature storage is permitted up to 1 month. Vials that have been frozen should be discarded. Before infusion, the product must be reconstituted according to the manufacturer's directions, using the diluent supplied or sterile water. PPC should not be refrigerated after reconstitution, but used immediately. Manufacturers recommend it be infused within 3 hours after reconstitution and any unused portion discarded.

Administration

The lyophilized product must be completely resuspended by gentle agitation or swirling before it is given intravenously. The common method of infusion is direct syringe injection. Manufacturers may supply a filter needle and recommend the resuspended product be filtered as the injection syringe is loaded. Several vials may be mixed into one syringe.

Infusion rates less than 10 ml/min are recommended. Vasomotor reactions have been reported with fast infusion rates.[98] Factor levels or coagulation studies should be evaluated following PCC therapy to assess its effectiveness.

Reactions

Rapid infusions of PCC have been associated with flushing, pulse increases and drops in blood pressure, presumably from the presence of vasoactive substances. Pyrogenic and allergic symptoms have also been reported: fever, chills, headache, flushing, tingling, urticaria, nausea, vomiting and general lethargy. These symptoms may disappear quickly when the infusion is stopped or slowed.[98]

Like Factor VIII concentrate, PCC exposes a patient to large numbers of donors and transmittable diseases such as hepatitis and AIDS. Heat-treated PCC is now produced by all manufacturers to reduce the risk of AIDS transmission and is considered the product of choice. However, PCC still carries a presumed risk of hepatitis.

Another complication of PCC is the development of serious thromboembolic episodes and/or DIC from the activated factors present.[75,83] Neonates, patients with liver disease, and hemophilia B patients receiving large, repetitive doses of PCC for major surgeries or crush injuries are especially vulnerable to these problems. The International Committee on Thrombosis and Haemostasis recommends adding heparin to PCC to a concentration of 2–5 units/ml to reduce this complication.[107] Any high-risk patient should be carefully monitored for signs or symptoms of intravascular coagulation or thrombosis during treatment.

Finally, anti-A and anti-B are present in PCC and may cause a positive DAT in patients who are group A, B or AB. Because of the risk of thrombosis and longer half-life of Factor IX, the quantities transfused are seldom large enough to cause apparent hemolysis. Myocardial infarctions have also been reported as a rare complication.[75] It has been proposed that the release of bradykinins following large repetitive doses leads to vascular leakage and myocardial injury.

Irradiated Blood Products

The subject of transfusion-associated graft-versus-host disease (GVHD) has been recently reviewed[108–110] and is summarized below from these references. GVHD can occur when functional, immunocompetent lymphocytes in a blood product engraft in a susceptible recipient and generate an immunological response against the host. GVHD following blood transfusion is similar to that seen postmarrow transplantation with fever, skin rash and gastrointestinal symptoms. However, acute transfusion-associated GVHD occurs much more rapidly (4–30 days posttransfusion) and is associated with profound bone marrow suppression. It almost never responds to therapy and, therefore, has a higher mortality rate.[109,110]

Patients at Risk

Patients at highest risk of developing GVHD include those with congenital cell-mediated immune defects such as severe combined immunodeficiency disease (SCID) or Wiskott-Aldrich syndrome.

Patients who have undergone allogeneic or autologous bone marrow transplantation are also at high risk because of the treatment they are given to eliminate malignant cells or permit engraftment of the new marrow. Patients at a lower and temporary risk are infants requiring intrauterine or exchange transfusions. It has been suggested that the fetal or neonatal immune system may be too immature to reject engraftment, or that intrauterine transfusions may induce a state of immune tolerance in the newborn. Patients with acute leukemia, Hodgkin's and non-Hodgkin's lymphomas, and children with neuroblastoma are also at some risk while they are immunosuppressed from their chemotherapy. Some patient groups do not appear to be susceptible to GVHD: those with solid tumors, aplastic anemia, agammaglobulinemia, chronic granulomatous disease, AIDS, and infants receiving standard blood transfusions.

Blood Components with Risk

Almost all blood components that have not been stored frozen have been implicated in transfusion-associated GVHD: whole blood, red cells, platelets, granulocytes, even fresh (not frozen) single donor plasma. All contain viable lymphocytes to a varying degree.[110] Granulocyte concentrates contain the greatest number, and, because they are given to patients with marrow hypoplasia and immune insufficiency, they put patients at increased risk. It is thought that a minimum dose of 1×10^7 lymphocytes/kg body weight is needed to induce GVHD, but this minimum may vary with the degree of immunodeficiency of the host. Three children with immunodeficiency disease developed GVHD after a dose of only 8×10^4 lymphocytes/kg from single transfusions of fresh single-donor plasma.[110]

Fresh frozen plasma and cryoprecipitate have not been associated with GVHD. These products do not contain cryoprotective agents to preserve any residual lymphocytes. Although deglycerolized red cells have also not been implicated in transfusion-associated GVHD, they contain $1–10 \times 10^7$ viable lymphocytes which could initiate a response.[109]

Prevention of GVHD

Irradiating blood products to 1500 rad effectively reduces the risk of transfusion-associated GVHD. Although levels as low as 500 rad completely abolish lymphocyte proliferation as measured by mixed lymphocyte culture, 1500 rad provide an extra margin of safety and do not adversely affect red cell, platelet or granulocyte function.[108]

Self-contained cesium-137 irradiators are most commonly used to irradiate blood products. Depending on the strength of the cesium source, 1–5 minutes may be needed to give a total dose of 1500 rad. Cobalt-60 therapy machines in the radiation therapy department may also be used, but these are less convenient and more expensive to operate, and require more time to make the arrangements.[109]

Selection and compatibility guidelines for irradiated blood products are the same as those for nonirradiated products. Irradiation does not change the product's expiration or storage requirements. No special precautions are needed during transfusion. These products are not "radioactive." If they are not used by the recipient for whom they were intended, they may be safely given to any patient, provided standard compatibility requirements are met.[109]

References

1. American Association of Blood Banks. American Red Cross, Council of Community Blood Centers. Circular of information for the use of human blood and blood products. Washington, DC: American Red Cross, October, 1984.
2. Snyder EL, ed. Blood transfusion therapy, a physician's handbook. Arlington, VA: American Association of Blood Banks, 1983.
3. Schmidt PJ, ed. Standards for blood banks and transfusion services. 11th ed. Arlington, VA: American Association of Blood Banks, 1984.
4. Widmann FK, ed. Technical manual. 9th ed. Arlington, VA: American Association of Blood Banks, 1985.
5. Jaffe ER. Erythrocyte metabolism and its relation to the liquid preservation of human blood. In: Petz LD, Swisher SN. Clinical practice of blood transfusion. London: Churchill Livingstone, 1981:265–87.
6. Schorr JB. Perinatal, neonatal and exchange transfusions. In: Mayer K, ed. Guidelines to transfusion practices. Washington, DC: American Association of Blood Banks, 1980:123–36.
7. Snyder EL, Bookbinder M. Role of microaggregate blood filtration in clinical medicine. Transfusion 1983;23:460–70.
8. Bowie EJW, Thompson JH, Owen CA. The stability of antihemophiliac globulin and labile factor in human blood. Mayo Clin Proc 1964;39:144–51.
9. Counts RB, Haisch C, Simon TL, Maxwell NG, Heimbach DM, Carrico CJ. Hemostasis in massively transfused trauma patients. Ann Surg 1979;190:91–9.

10. Latham JT, Bove JR, Weirich FL. Chemical and hematologic changes in stored CPDA-1 blood. Transfusion 1982;22:158–9.

11. Moore GL, Peck CC, Sohmer PR, Zuck TF. Some properties of blood stored in anticoagulant CPDA-1 solution. Transfusion 1981;21:135–7.

12. Beutler E, Wood L. The in vivo regeneration of red cell 2,3-diphosphoglyceric acid (DPG) after transfusion of stored blood. J Lab Clin Med 1969;74:300–4.

13. Friedman BA. An analysis of surgical blood use in United States hospitals with application to the maximum surgical blood order schedule. Transfusion 1979;19:168–78.

14. Meryman HT, Bross J, Lebovitz R. The preparation of leukocyte-poor red blood cells: A comparative study. Transfusion 1980;20:285–92.

15. Wenz B, Gurtlinger KF, O'Toole AM, Dugan EP. Preparation of granulocyte-poor red blood cells by microaggregate filtration: A simplified method to minimize febrile transfusion reactions. Vox Sang 1980;39:282–7.

16. Parravicini A, Rebulla P, Apuzzo J, Wenz B, Sirchia G. The preparation of leukocyte-poor red cells for transfusion by a simple cost-effective technique. Transfusion 1984;24:508–9.

17. Menitove JE, McElligott MC, Aster RH. Febrile transfusion reactions: What blood component should be given next? Vox Sang 1982;42:318–21.

18. Mollison PL. Blood transfusion in clinical medicine. 7th ed. Oxford: Blackwell Scientific Publications, 1983:740.

19. Sherman SP, Taswell HF. The need for transfusion of saline-washed red blood cells to patients with paroxysmal nocturnal hemoglobinuria: a myth. Transfusion 1977;17:683 (abstract).

20. Jenkins DE. Paroxysmal nocturnal hemoglobinuria hemolytic systems. In: Bell C, ed. A seminar on laboratory management of hemolysis. Washington, DC: American Association of Blood Banks, 1979:45–69.

21. Meryman HT. Cryopreservation of blood and marrow cells; basic biological and biophysical considerations. In: Petz LD, Swisher SN. Clinical practice of blood transfusion. London: Churchill Livingstone, 1981:313–31.

22. Opelz G, Terasaki PI. Dominant effect of transfusions on kidney graft survival. Transplantation 1980;29:153–8.

23. Myhre BA. Quality control in blood banking. New York: John Wiley & Sons, 1974:168.

24. Butch S. Laboratory aspects of transfusion. In: Barnes A, Nelson IF, eds. Safe transfusion. Washington, DC: American Association of Blood Banks, 1981:33–45.

25. Luban NLC. Mechanical devices in pediatric transfusion. In: Luban NLC, Kolins J, eds. Hemotherapy in childhood and adolescence. Arlington, VA: American Association of Blood Banks, 1985:69–99.

26. Gibson JS, Leff RD, Roberts RJ. Effects of intravenous delivery systems on infused red blood cells. Am J Hosp Pharm 1984;41:468–72.

27. Kevy SV. Guidelines for blood ordering. In: Luban NLC, Kolins J, eds. Hemotherapy in childhood and adolescence. Arlington, VA: American Association of Blood Banks 1985:1–13.

28. Gianino N. Equipment used for transfusion. In: Rutman RC, Miller WV, eds. Transfusion therapy principles and procedures. 2nd ed. Rockville, MD: Aspen Systems Corporation, 1985:147–67.

29. Brady MT, Milan JD, Anderson DC, et al. Use of deglycerolized red blood cells to prevent posttransfusion infection with cytomegalovirus. J Infect Dis 1984;150:334–9.

30. Tomasulo PA, Lenes BA. Platelet transfusion therapy. In: Menitove JE, McCarthy LJ, eds. Hemostatic disorders and the blood bank. Arlington, VA: American Association of Blood Banks, 1984:63–89.

31. Simpson MB. Platelet function and transfusion therapy in the surgical patient. In: Schiffer CJ, ed. Platelet physiology and transfusion. Washington, DC: American Association of Blood Banks, 1978:51–67.

32. Slichter SJ, Harker LA. Thrombocytopenia: mechanisms and management of defects in platelet production. Clin Haematol 1978;7:523–39.

33. Silvergleid AJ. Clinical platelet transfusions. In: Silver H, ed. Blood, blood components and derivatives in transfusion therapy. Washington, DC: American Association of Blood Banks, 1980:45–88.

34. Westphal RG. Disseminated intravascular coagulation. In: Menitove JE, McCarthy LJ, eds. Hemostatic disorders and the blood bank. Arlington, VA: American Association of Blood Banks, 1984:25–39.

35. Champion AB, Carmen RA. Factors affecting white cell content in platelet concentrates. Transfusion 1985;25:334–8.

36. Simon TL, Henderson R. Coagulation factor activity in platelet concentrates. Transfusion 1979;19:186–9.

37. Menitove JE, Aster RH. Transfusion of platelets and plasma products. Clin Haematol 1983;12:239.

38. Schoendorfer DW, Hansen LE, Kenney DM. The surge technique: A method to increase purity of platelet concentrates

obtained by centrifugal apheresis. Transfusion 1983;23:182–9.

39. Schiffer CA, Slichter SJ. Platelet transfusions from single donors. N Engl J Med 1982;307:245–7.

40. Slichter SJ. Optimum platelet concentrate preparation and storage. In: Garratty G, ed. Current concepts in transfusion therapy. Arlington, VA: American Association of Blood Banks, 1985:1–26.

41. Murphy S, Gardner FH. Platelet preservation. Effect of storage temperature on maintenance of platelet viability—deleterious effect of refrigerated storage. N Engl J Med 1969; 280:1094–8.

42. Butch SH. Technical aspects of transfusion. In: Luban NLC, Keating LJ, eds. Hemotherapy of the infant and premature. Arlington, VA: American Association of Blood Banks, 1983:95–127.

43. Herzig RH, Herzig GP, Bull MI, et al. Correction of poor platelet transfusion responses with leukocyte-poor HLA-matched platelet concentrates. Blood 1975; 46:743–50.

44. Medeiros J, Dzik W. Leuko-poor platelet concentrates: A direct comparison of three blood filters. Ann Clin Lab Sc 1985;15:237–40.

45. Silvergleid AJ, Hafleigh EB, Harabin MA, Wolf RM, Grumet FC. Clinical value of washed platelet concentrates in patients with non-hemolytic transfusion reactions. Transfusion 1976;17:33–7.

46. Goldfinger D, McGinnis MH. Rh incompatible platelet transfusions— risks and consequences of sensitizing immunosuppressed patients. N Engl J Med 1971;284:942–9.

47. Arora SN, Morse EE. Platelet filters—an evaluation. Transfusion 1972;12:208–10.

48. Snyder EL, Ferri PM, Smith EO, Ezekowitz MD. Use of mechanical infusion pump for transfusion of platelet concentrates. Transfusion 1984;24:524–7.

49. Crosson JT. Blood component therapy. In: Marnette BL, Brzica SM, eds. From vein to vein, a seminar for phlebotomists and transfusionists. Washington, DC: American Association of Blood Banks, 1976:15–22.

50. Moroff G, Robkin-Kline L, Friedman A, Luban NLC. Procedures for the transfusion of platelets to newborns. Transfusion 1983; 23:431 (abstract).

51. Howard JE, Perkins HA. The natural history of alloimmunization to platelets. Transfusion 1978;18:496–503.

52. Higby DJ, Burnett, D. Granulocyte transfusions: Current status. Blood 1980;55:2–8.

53. Winston DJ, Ho WG, Gale RP. Therapeutic granulocyte transfusions for documented infections. Ann Intern Med 1982;97:509–15.

54. Herzig RH. Granulocyte transfusion therapy: Past, present and future. In: Garratty G, ed. Current concepts in transfusion therapy. Arlington, VA: American Association of Blood Banks, 1985:267–94.

55. Boggs DR. The kinetics of neutrophil leukocytes in health and disease. Sem in Hematol 1967;4:359–86.

56. Higby DJ. Granulocyte transfusions. In: Silver H, ed. Blood, blood components and derivatives in transfusion therapy. Washington, DC: American Association of Blood Banks, 1980:29–44.

57. Christensen RD, Anstall HB, Rothstein G. Review: Deficiencies in the neutrophil system of newborn infants, and the use of leukocyte transfusions in the treatment of neonatal sepsis. J Clin Apheresis 1982;1:33–41.

58. Christensen RD, Anstall HB, Rothstein G. Depletion of neutrophil during neonatal septicemia: Mechanisms involved and experimental treatment. In: Luban NLC, Keating LJ, eds. Hemotherapy of the infant and premature. Arlington, VA: American Association of Blood Banks, 1983:51–68.

59. Laurenti F, Ferro R, Isacch G, et al. Polymorphonuclear leukocyte transfusions for the treatment of sepsis in the newborn infant. J Pediatr 1981;98:118–23.

60. Nusbacher J, MacPherson J. A comparison of technics for leukopheresis and platelet pheresis. In: Nusbacher J, Berkman EM, eds. Fundamentals of a pheresis program. Washington, DC: American Association of Blood Banks, 1979;49–61.

61. Rock G, Zurakowski S, Baxter A, Adams G. Simple and rapid preparation of granulocytes for the treatment of neonatal septicemia. Transfusion 1984;24:510–2.

62. Goldfinger D, Medici MA, Hsi R, McPherson J, Connelly M. Preparation and in vitro function of granulocyte concentrates for transfusion to neonates using the IBM 2991 blood processor. Transfusion 1983;23:358–60.

63. McCullough J, Weiblen BJ, Fine D. Effects of storage of granulocytes on their fate in vivo. Transfusion 1983;23:20–4.

64. McCullough J, Weiblen BJ, Peterson PK, Quie PG. Effects of temperature on granulocyte preservation. Blood 1987;52:301–10.

65. Richman CM. Prolonged cryopreservation of human granulocytes. Transfusion 1983;23:508–11.

66. Clay ME, Kline WE. Detection of granulocyte antigens and antibodies: Current perspectives and approaches. In: Gar-

ratty G, ed. Current concepts in transfusion therapy. Arlington, VA: American Association of Blood Banks, 1985:183–266.

67. Snyder EL, Root RK, Hezzey A, Metcalf J, Palermo G. Effect of microaggregate blood filtration on granulocyte concentrates in vitro. Transfusion 1983;23:25–9.

68. Christensen RD, Anstall H, Rothstein G. Neutrophil transfusion in septic neutropenic neonates. Transfusion 1982;22:151–3.

69. Consensus development panel, National Institutes of Health. Fresh frozen plasma: indications and risks. JAMA 1985;253:551–3.

70. Braunstein AH, Oberman HA. Transfusion of plasma components. Transfusion 1984;24:281–6.

71. Oberman HA. Uses and abuses of fresh frozen plasma. In: Garratty G, ed. Current concepts in transfusion therapy. Arlington, VA: American Association of Blood Banks, 1985:109–24.

72. Aronson DL. Factor IX complex. Semin Thromb Hemost 1979;6:28–43.

73. Counts RB. Acquired bleeding disorders. In: Menitove JE, McCarthy LJ, eds. Hemostatic disorders and the blood bank. Arlington, VA: American Association of Blood Banks, 1984:41–7.

74. Cartun SM, Snyder EL. Thrombotic disorders: A clinical review. In: Menitove JE, McCarthy LJ, eds. Hemostatic disorders and the blood bank. Arlington, VA: American Association of Blood Banks, 1984:91–118.

75. Lusher JM. Replacement therapy for congenital and acquired disorders of blood coagulation—available products. In: Garratty G, ed. Current concepts in transfusion therapy. Arlington, VA: American Association of Blood Banks, 1985:27–49.

76. Toy PT, Johnston C. Therapeutic apheresis in hematological diseases. In: Kolins J, Jones JM, eds. Therapeutic apheresis. Arlington, VA: American Association of Blood Banks, 1983:89–97.

77. Breckenridge RL, Solberg LA, Pineda AA, Petitt RM, Dharkar DD. Treatment of thrombocytopenic purpura with plasma exchange, antiplatelet agent, corticosteroid, and plasma infusion: Mayo clinic experience. J Clin Apheresis 1982;1:6–13.

78. Wintrobe MM, Lee GR, Boggs DR, et al. Clinical hematology. 8th ed. Philadelphia: Lea & Febinger, 1981:1185.

79. Rizza ER. Management of patients with inherited blood coagulation defects. In: Bloom AL, Thomas DP, eds. Hemostasis and thrombosis. London: Churchill Livingstone, 1981:371.

80. Kennedy MS, Adkins S, Wansky J. Blood components. In: Barnes A, Nelson I, eds. Safe transfusion. Washington, DC: American Association of Blood Banks, 1981:1–13.

81. Kevy SV, Fosburg M, Wolfe L. The use of platelets, plasma and plasma derivatives in the newborn. In: Luban NLC, Keating LJ, eds. Hemotherapy of the infant and premature. Arlington, VA: American Association of Blood Banks, 1983:37–50.

82. Snyder EL, Ferri PM, Mosher DF. Fibronectin in liquid and frozen stored blood components. Transfusion 1984;24:53–6.

83. Kasper CK. Hematologic treatment of hemophilia and von Willebrand disease. In: Luban NLC, Kolins J, eds. Hemotherapy in childhood and adolescence. Arlington, VA: American Association of Blood Banks, 1985:53–68.

84. Zimmerman TS, Ruggeri MA. Von Willebrand's disease. Prog Hemost Thromb 1982;6:203–36.

85. Williams WJ. Congenital deficiency of Factor XIII (fibrin-stabilizing factor). In: Williams WJ, Beutler E, Erslev AJ, Rundles RW. Hematology. 2nd ed. New York: McGraw-Hill Book Company, 1977:1431–3.

86. Mosher DF. Fibronectin—relevance to hemostasis and thrombosis. In: Colman RW, Hirsh J, Marder VJ, Salzman EW, eds. Hemostasis and thrombosis: Basic principles and clinical practice. Philadelphia: JB Lippincott Company, 1982:174–84.

87. Gandhi JG, Vander Salm T, Szymanski IO. Effect of cardiopulmonary bypass on plasma fibronectin, IgG, and C3. Transfusion 1983;23:476–9.

88. Saba TM, Blumenstock FA, Scovill WA, Bernard H. Cryoprecipitate reversal of opsonic α 2SB glycoprotein deficiency in septic surgical and trauma patients. Science 1978;201:622–4.

89. Saba TM, Blumenstock FA, Weber P, Kaplan JE. Physiologic role for cold-insoluble globulin in systemic host defense: Implications of its characterization as the opsonic α 2SB glycoprotein. Ann NY Acad Sci 1978;312:43–55.

90. Janson PA, Jubelirer SJ, Weinstein MJ, Deykin D. Treatment of the bleeding tendency in uremia with cryoprecipitate. N Engl J Med 1980;303:1318–22.

91. Gerritsen SW, Akkerman JWN, Sixma JJ. Correction of the bleeding time in patients with storage pool deficiency by infusion of cryoprecipitate. Br J Haematol 1978;40:153–60.

92. Sherer JF. Cryoprecipitate coagulum pyelolithotomy. J Urol 1980;123:621–4.

93. Fischer CP, Sonda LP, Dionko AC. Use of cryoprecipitate coagulum in extracting renal calculi. Urol 1980;15:6–13.

94. Inwood MJ, Barr JD, Warren BA, Chauvin WJ. Filtration of cryoprecipitate: a microscopic assessment of filter deposition. Transfusion 1978;18:722–7.

95. Britten AFH. Plasma procurement and fractionation: A worldwide overview. In: Kolins J, Britten AFH, Silvergleid AJ, eds. Plasma products: Use and management. Arlington, VA: American Association of Blood Banks, 1982:1–22.

96. Snyder EL. Clinical use of albumin, plasma protein fraction and isoimmune globulin products. In: Kolins J, Britten AFH, Silvergleid AJ, eds. Plasma products: use and management. Arlington, VA: American Association of Blood Banks, 1982:87–107.

97. Silver H. Normal serum albumin and plasma protein fraction. In: Silver H, ed. Blood, blood components and derivatives in transfusion therapy. Washington, DC: American Association of Blood Banks, 1980:89–95.

98. Boyd JR, Olin BR, Hunsaker LM, eds. Facts and comparisons (with monthly updates). St. Louis, MO: JB Lippincott Company, 1984.

99. Brown WJ, Kim BS, Weeks DB, Parkin CE. Physiologic saline solution, Normosol R pH 7.4 and Plasmanate as reconstituents of packed human erythrocytes. Anesthesiology 1978;49:99–101.

100. Piszkiewicz D, Kingdom H, Apfelzweig R, et al. Inactivation of HTLV-III/LAV during plasma fractionation (letter). Lancet 1985;2:1188–9.

101. Kelton JG. The interaction of IgG with reticuloendothelial cells: Biological and therapeutic implications. In: Garratty G, ed. Current concepts in transfusion therapy. Arlington, VA: American Association of Blood Banks, 1985:51–107.

102. Lang GE, Veldhuis B. Immune serum globulin—a cause of anti-Rh₀ (D) passive sensitization. Am J Clin Pathol 1973; 60:205–7.

103. Lever AML, Brown D, Webster ADB, Thomas HC. Non-A,non-B hepatitis occurring in agammaglobulinemic patients after intravenous immunoglobulin. Lancet 1984;2:1062–3.

104. National Hemophilia Foundation's Medical and Scientific Advisory Council. Recommendations concerning AIDS and therapy of hemophilia (revised March 1, 1985). New York: National Hemophilia Foundation, 1985.

105. Boese EC, Tantum KR, Eyster ME. Pulmonary function abnormalities after infusion of antihemophilic factor (AHF) concentrates. Am J Med 1979;67:474–6.

106. Gerety RJ, Eyster ME, Tabor E, et al. Hepatitis B virus, hepatitis A virus and persistently elevated amino transferases in hemophiliacs. J Med Virol 1980;6:111–8.
107. Menache D, Roberts HR. Summary report and recommendation of task force members and consultants. Thrombos Diath Haemorrh 1975;33:645–7.
108. Leitman SF, Holland PV. Irradiation of blood products—indications and guidelines. Transfusion 1985;25:293–303.
109. Holland PV. Transfusion-associated graft-versus-host disease: Prevention using irradiated blood products. In: Garratty G, ed. Current concepts in transfusion therapy. Arlington, VA: American Association of Blood Banks, 1985:295–315.
110. Leitman SF. Posttransfusion graft-versus-host disease. In: Smith DM, Silvergleid AJ, eds. Special considerations in transfusing the immunocompromised patient. Arlington, VA: American Association of Blood Banks, 1985:15–37.

Appendix 3-1. A Summary of ABO/Rh Compatibility

I. Antigens and Antibodies

	Blood Group	Antigens on Red Blood Cells	Antibodies in Serum
ABO	A	A	Anti-B
	B	B	Anti-A
	AB	A and B	—
	O	—	Anti-A and Anti-B
Rh	Rh-pos	D	—
	Rh-neg	—	Anti-D *only* if sensitized

II. Blood Product Compatibility

Whole Blood —Must be ABO-identical to patient.

Red Blood Cells —Must be compatible with patient serum.

Platelets —Should be compatible with patient red cells. Any blood group may be given if need is urgent.

Granulocytes —Should be compatible with patient serum.

Plasma —Should be compatible with patient red cells.

Cryoprecipitate —Should be compatible with patient red cells. Any blood group may be given if need is urgent.

If the patient is:	Blood Group Compatible with Patient Serum	Blood Group Compatible with Patient Cells
A	A, O	A, AB
B	B, O	B, AB
AB	AB, A, B, O	AB only
O	O only	O, A, B, AB
Rh-pos	Rh-pos and Rh-neg	(Rh not considered)
Rh-neg	Rh-neg	(Rh not considered)

In: Reynolds, AW and Steckler, D, eds.
Practical Aspects of Blood Administration
Arlington, VA: American Association
of Blood Banks, 1986

4

Adverse Effects of Blood Transfusion

Margie B. Peschel, MD

*A*DVERSE EFFECTS OF BLOOD transfusion possibly date back to 1492. There is an apocryphal story that, when Pope Innocent VIII was on his deathbed, a last desperate attempt at his revival was made on the recommendation of an unknown physician. He received blood from three youths and, shortly thereafter, he passed on, doubtlessly to Heaven. So did the three youths, one hopes. The prescribing physician wisely and quickly disappeared, in which direction is not recorded.[1]

Every transfusion of blood or one of its components is followed by a "transfusion reaction." The reaction, in most instances, is a beneficial one, manifested by a favorable response of the patient in need of blood or blood component to correct a deficit. In a small number (0.5-3%) [2(p 738–9)-5] of transfusions, the response is not as expected, and the recipient experiences an adverse effect. Adverse effects may occur during and following transfusion. Delayed reactions and disease transmission may not be manifested until days, months or years after transfusion. Most adverse effects are totally unexpected and unpreventable, but some can be prevented. Adverse effects of blood transfusion vary from being relatively benign to lethal. In view of the potential for serious adverse reactions in every transfused patient, knowledgeable medical supervision, close observation of qualified nursing staff and prompt evaluation by laboratory staff are necessary for safe transfusion.

Signs and Symptoms of Adverse Effects

Immediate adverse effects of blood transfusion are manifested by a variety of clinical signs and symptoms. These include chills, fever, flushing, pruritus, urticaria, dyspnea, back or chest pain, hemoglo-

Margie B. Peschel, MD, Medical Director, Carter Blood Center, Fort Worth, Texas

binuria, shock and generalized bleeding. The time that elapses between signs and symptoms and initiation of appropriate therapy must be as short as possible. Delayed reactions are more subtle and often missed. Information and instructions to follow regarding adverse reactions must be in every facility's procedures manual.

Immediate Adverse Reactions

Acute Hemolytic Transfusion Reactions (AHTR)

The most lethal complication of blood transfusions is destruction of donor red cells triggered by an antigen-antibody reaction. The most serious hemolytic reactions involve ABO incompatibility, but other antibodies which bind complement and possess lytic properties such as anti-Kidd[a] and less commonly anti-Kell, anti-P and anti-Duffy[a], may infrequently cause a less severe hemolytic reaction. Most AHTR are preventable and are the result of a clerical error with misidentification of patient, sample or unit of blood. The onset of fever and shaking chills alerts one to the probability of an acute hemolytic transfusion reaction. Hemoglobinuria, hemoglobinemia, fall in blood pressure and rapid pulse may all be demonstrable. The direct antiglobulin test (DAT) on the posttransfusion specimen is positive and the offending antibody can be eluted from the red cells.[5]

When donor red cells with A and B antigens on their surface are transfused into a recipient with anti-A or anti-B in the plasma, interaction of antibody with antigen initiates activation of three biological systems (complement, kinin and coagulation).

Activation of complement produces holes in the surface membranes of red cells, leading to their destruction or acute intravascular hemolysis. Both free hemoglobin and red cell stroma enter the plasma. Free hemoglobin was formerly thought to play a major role in renal ischemia, but current thought is that the antibody-coated cell stroma contributes to renal vasoconstriction. Activation of complement also results in anaphylatoxic stimulation of mast cells, which release serotinin and histamine, producing a fall in blood pressure and shock.

Activation of kinins produces a neuroendocrine response with the sympathetic nervous system and adrenal glands pouring out norepinephrine and other catecholamines, which act on alpha receptors in blood vessels, causing intense vasoconstriction of the renal, splanchnic, pulmonary and cutaneous capillaries.

Antigen-antibody complexes can activate the coagulation system with formation of small clots in the circulation, a process known as disseminated intravascular coagulation (DIC). The cumulative effect may end in acute renal failure or uncontrollable shock.[6, 7]

The mainstays of therapy for AHTR are the maintenance of blood pressure and renal blood flow. If shock can be prevented or adequately treated, renal failure can usually be avoided. Fluid therapy should be directed at maintaining urine flow over 100 ml/hr for at least 24 hours. To improve blood flow to kidneys and increase urine output 20–80 mg, IV furosemide (Lasix) will increase the renal blood flow and produce a diuresis.[8] Mannitol 20 g in 250 ml of saline intravenously (an osmotic diuretic) will increase urine flow but does not necessarily improve renal perfusion. Vasopressor agents that decrease renal blood flow are contraindicated. Dopamine hydrochloride may be very useful in treating shock associated with AHTR because it dilates renal vasculature while increasing cardiac output. DIC with resulting bleeding is in some instances the predominant problem. Heparin therapy of DIC is controversial and is probably only indicated when the reaction is due to ABO mismatch and the patient has received more than 200 ml of blood. A dose of 5000 units of heparin IV followed by IV infusion of 1500 units each hour for 6–24 hours has been recommended. In the patient with exposed surgical field or extensive trauma, heparinization is probably too risky.[8] Death from incompatible transfusions is rare today, due to prompt recognition and management of this life-threatening adverse effect of transfusion.

Nonimmunologic Causes of Hemolysis

Hemolysis can occur during or following transfusion from reasons other than antigen-antibody reactions. In the absence of serological evidence of incompatibility, investigation must proceed immediately to determine cause for hemoglobinuria and hemoglobinemia. Possible causes include: 1) overheating in blood warmer, 2) blood storage at too low a temperature, 3) concurrent infusion of nonisotonic solutions with osmotic lysis of red cells, 4) mechanical trauma from faulty equipment, such as a pump oxygenator, 5) infusion under pressure through a small needle, 6) unrecognized paroxysmal nocturnal hemoglobinuria, 7) G6PD deficiency, 8) Sickle cell crisis and 9) sepsis (Clostridium perfringens in patient or contaminated blood).

Febrile Nonhemolytic Reactions (FNHR)

FNHR is the most common adverse effect of transfusion. The problem with FNHR is that it cannot be differentiated from early stages of AHTR. A febrile nonhemolytic reaction is a temperature rise of 1 C or more occurring in association with transfusion and without other explanation. The patient usually has a history of many transfusions or pregnancies. The vast majority are probably attributable to leukoagglutinins or platelet agglutinins. The cause of others remains obscure. When a febrile reaction occurs, transfusion is stopped, venous access maintained, a clerical check performed and blood bank notified. The procedure for AHTR is followed until blood bank reports that investigation is negative for incompatibility or hemolysis.[9] Fever may be mild to severe and usually responds to antipyretics. FNHR can be prevented by leucocyte-poor saline washed red cells or microaggregate filtration.[10, 11] This is usually recommended after two or more FNHR.

Allergic Reactions

Urticarial allergic reactions are characterized by hives, local erythema and itching and is the second most frequently encountered adverse effect of transfusion. Transfusion is interrupted and an antihistamine (50 mg diphenhydramine IM) is administered. After relief of symptoms, the transfusion may be continued slowly. Recipients who have frequent urticarial reactions may be pretreated with antihistamines or given washed red blood cells.[12] The etiology is unknown.

A rare severe anaphylactic reaction may occur after infusion of only a few milliliters of blood or plasma. It is characterized by rapid onset of acute respiratory distress, cyanosis and shock. Most of these reactions occur in IgA-deficient patients who have developed anti-IgA antibodies. Treatment is to stop transfusion and give epinephrine. Deglycerolized red cells or autologous transfusion may be used for further red cell transfusion. Components that contain plasma must be from IgA-deficient donors. Following an anaphylactic reaction, quantitative immunoglobulin and presence or absence of IgA antibodies should be ascertained. Individuals who are both IgA deficient and who have anti-IgA antibodies (high titered) should be informed and advised to wear a Medic-Alert bracelet.

Circulatory Overload

Circulatory overload occurs in infants, elderly, severely anemic and cardiac patients. Symptoms include coughing, cyanosis and difficulty in breathing, which reflect developing pulmonary edema. If circulatory overload is suspected, stop the transfusion, place the patient in a sitting position, and administer diuretics and oxygen.

Patients susceptible to circulatory overload should receive only red cells, not whole blood, and small volumes slowly infused.

Bacterial Contamination

Septicemia from blood results in chills, fever and decreased blood pressure ("red shock"), and measures must be instituted at once to save the patient. Gram stain of donor blood or component is often sufficient to establish diagnosis. Culture of the blood is usually gram-negative bacilli. Treatment is immediate, consisting of IV antibiotics combined with treatment for shock.[2(p 729–80), 13]

Noncardiogenic Pulmonary Edema

This exceedingly rare reaction seems confined to the lungs. Symptoms include shortness of breath, cyanosis and decreased blood pressure with pulmonary edema findings. Apparently, it is caused by donor leukoagglutinins and recipient leukocytes producing white cell aggregates that are trapped in pulmonary circulation. The treatment is to stop the transfusion and give steroids and respiratory support. This severe reaction may result in death.

Delayed Reactions

Delayed reactions include delayed hemolytic transfusion reactions and infectious complications. In contrast to AHTR, delayed hemolytic transfusion reactions (DHTR), for the most part, and infectious complications are not preventable.

Delayed Hemolytic Transfusion Reactions

The patients usually have a compatible crossmatch and receive a unit of blood. Most cases are subclinical, but a triad of fever, anemia and recent transfusion deserves investigation. A common denominator for all is that the patient has been either previously transfused or pregnant. The antibodies most likely to produce DHTR are anti-Kidd, Duffy, Kell, E, c and D. The antibody is not evident by laboratory tests but the patient's antibody system has been primed to react against that antigen. If the patient is then transfused with the antigen on the red cell, the primed antibody system will produce antibody rapidly. The cells are removed by macrophages, with the end result that 4 to 21 days after transfusion, the transfused red cells are destroyed. The anemia that results may prompt requests for more blood. A positive direct antiglobulin test will result and an antibody not present on the previous crossmatch will be detected. Patients who develop significant antibodies should be informed and an appropriate notation made in medical records to avoid hemolytic reactions during subsequent transfusions.[5]

Viral Hepatitis

Transfusion-associated hepatitis (TAH) remains a most serious complication of blood transfusion. The onset, which usually occurs from 90–180 days after transfusion, may occur anytime between 14 days and about 9 months. Hepatitis B has been significantly reduced by third generation testing for HBsAg and by volunteer (rather than paid) blood donation. Transmission of type A virus by transfusion is extremely rare, because there is apparently no viremia or carrier state of this virus. However, a previously unsuspected virus (or perhaps several viruses) has emerged as the most common cause of TAH. The etiologic agent for at least 90% of TAH has been termed non-A,non-B hepatitis. Prevention depends on careful screening of donors and careful follow-up of recipients to detect TAH. Physicians should be aware of the necessity of reporting all cases of suspected TAH.

Malaria

Malaria is a very rare complication. Exclusion of donors at high risk is the only effective preventive measure.

Syphilis

The risk of syphilis is small. Treponema cannot survive at refrigeration temperatures. Serologic testing of donor blood is no longer required by the AABB *Standards*, but is required by federal regulation.

Cytomegalovirus

Cytomegalovirus (CMV) has been implicated in "posttransfusion" syndrome, an infectious mononucleosis-like condition occurring after open heart surgery. Cytomegalovirus has also been implicated in posttransfusion hepatitis. CMV is a member of the herpes virus group. The virus lies dormant in healthy individuals and is carried in leukocytes. Cytomegalovirus may be transmitted if blood infected with CMV is transfused. Infection depends on the immune state of the recipient, and recent CMV infections have been reported to occur in immunosuppressed patients. Cytomegalovirus presents a problem to the neonatal patient and may be fatal if the child weighs less than 1200 grams. If the infant weighs over 1200 grams, the infant may be asymptomatic or have respiratory problems.

Acquired Immune Deficiency Syndrome (AIDS)

Fewer than 2% of the reported AIDS cases have been thought to be transmitted by blood transfusion. Even this risk will be virtually eliminated with the application of the HTLV-III antibody test, coupled with continued use of self-exclusion criteria for high risk groups. However, because the incubation period for AIDS can be more than 5 years, new cases of transfusion-associated AIDS can be expected to appear for some time in persons infected with HTLV-III virus before the blood screening test came into use in 1985.[14]

Graft-Versus-Host Disease

Graft-versus-host disease (GVHD) occurs in patients receiving bone marrow transplant and very rarely in transfused patient being extensively treated with chemotherapy and irradiation. Clinical syndrome of GVHD includes fever, skin rash, hepatitis and diarrhea. Preirradiation of blood components containing lymphocytes prevents GVHD.

Hemosiderosis

Every unit of red cells contains 250 milligrams of iron. When long-term transfusion is required, iron deposition can occur and interfere with the function of the heart, liver and endocrine glands. Preventive treatment is the use of fresh red cells and/or iron chelating agents.

Conclusion

The basic principle in transfusion therapy is "*primum non nocere—first do no harm.*" Though transfusion fatality rate is small, deaths do occur. ABO hemolytic reactions due to clerical errors remain the most serious problem. Careful observation of symptoms, clinical signs and appropriate laboratory evaluation of adverse effects of transfusion result in safe transfusion practices.

References

1. Diamond L. A history of blood transfusion. In: Wintrobe M, ed. Blood, pure and eloquent. New York: McGraw-Hill, 1980:660.
2. Mollison PL. Some unfavorable effects of transfusions. In: Blood transfusion in clinical medicine. 7th ed. Oxford: Blackwell Scientific, 1983:738–9.
3. Myhre B. Fatalities from blood transfusion. JAMA 1980;224:1333–5.
4. Schmidt P. Transfusion reactions. Clin Lab Med 1982;2:221–31.
5. Taswell H, Pineda A, Moore SB. Hemolytic transfusion reactions: Frequency and clinical and laboratory aspects. In: Bell C, ed. A seminar on immune-mediated cell destruction. Washington, DC: American Association of Blood Banks, 1981:71–92.
6. Barnes A. Complications of transfusion. In: Barnes A, Nelson I, ed. Safe transfusion. Washington, DC: American Association of Blood Banks, 1981:63–76.
7. Widmann FK, ed. Technical manual. 9th ed. Arlington, VA: American Association of Blood Banks, 1985:325–344.
8. Goldfinger D. Acute hemolytic transfusion reactions—a fresh look at pathogenesis and considerations regarding therapy. Transfusion 1977;17:85–98.
9. McCord R, Myhre B. A method for rapid and thorough workup of febrile and allergic transfusion reactions. Lab Med 1978;9:39–46.
10. Schned A, Silver H. The use of microaggregate filtration in the prevention of febrile transfusion reactions. Transfusion 1981;21:675–81.
11. Meryman H, McCullough J. The preparation of red cells depleted of leukocytes: Review and evaluation. Transfusion 1986;26:101–6.
12. Goldfinger D, Lowe IC. Prevention of adverse reactions to blood transfusion by administration of saline-washed red blood cells. Transfusion 1981;21:277–80.
13. Arnon P, Weiss L. Escherichia Coli sepsis from contaminated platelet transfusion. Ann Intern Med 1986;146:321–4.
14. Centers for Disease Control: Update—AIDS. MMWR 1985;34:245–8.

Index